Medicine and moral reasoning

Medicine and moral reasoning

Edited by K. W. M. Fulford
Research Fellow, Green College, University of Oxford

Grant R. Gillett
Associate Professor of Medical Ethics, University of Otago

and Janet Martin Soskice
University Lecturer, Faculty of Divinity, University of Cambridge

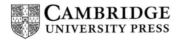
CAMBRIDGE
UNIVERSITY PRESS

Published by the Press Syndicate of the University of Cambridge
The Pitt Building, Trumpington Street, Cambridge CB2 1RP
40 West 20th Street, New York, NY 10011–4211, USA
10 Stamford Road, Oakleigh, Melbourne 3166, Australia

First published 1994

Printed in Great Britain at the University Press, Cambridge

A catalogue record for this book is available from the British Library

Library of Congress cataloguing in publication data

Medicine and moral reasoning/edited by K. W. M. Fulford, Grant R.
Gillett, and Janet Martin Soskice.
   p. cm.
Includes index.
ISBN 0 521 45325 9 (hardback)
1. Medical ethics. 2. Judgement (Ethics). I. Fulford, K. W. M.
II. Gillett, Grant R. III. Soskice, Janet Martin.
[DNLM: 1. Ethics, Medical. 2. Morals. W 50 M48975 1994]
R724.M2993   1994
174′.2–dc20
DNLM/DLC
93-10595CIP

ISBN 0 521 45325 9 hardback
ISBN 0 521 45946 X paperback

Contents

Contributors

JASON BRANDT Associate Professor of Psychiatry, Department of Psychiatry and Behavioral Sciences, Johns Hopkins Medical Institutions, USA

ALASTAIR V. CAMPBELL Professor of Medical Ethics, Bioethics Research Centre, University of Otago, New Zealand

ROGER CRISP Fellow, St Anne's College, University of Oxford

K. WILLIAM M. FULFORD Research Fellow, Green College, University of Oxford

GRANT R. GILLETT Associate Professor of Medical Ethics, Bioethics Research Centre, University of Otago, New Zealand

MIRIAM GRIFFIN Fellow and Tutor in Ancient History, Somerville College, University of Oxford

RICHARD M. HARE Professor of Philosophy, University of Florida, USA

MICHAEL LOCKWOOD Tutor in Philosophy, Department of External Studies, University of Oxford

WILLIAM F. MAY Professor of Biomedical Ethics, Southern Methodist University, Galveston, USA

MARY MIDGLEY Formerly Senior Lecturer in Philosophy, University of Newcastle-on-Tyne

THOMAS H. MURRAY Director, Center for Biomedical Ethics, Case Western Reserve University, USA

GRAHAM ODDIE Professor of Philosophy, Massey University, New Zealand

JANET M. SOSKICE Fellow, Jesus College, University of Cambridge

JAMES O. URMSON Emeritus Professor, Stanford University; Emeritus Fellow, Corpus Christi College, University of Oxford

Acknowledgements

The editors are grateful to Mrs Caroline Miles and the Rev. Dr A. R. Peacocke for their encouragement and support during the preparation of this volume. A number of the contributions are based on seminars held at the Ian Ramsey Centre, St Cross College, Oxford.

Professor R. M. Hare's contribution has appeared previously in *Bioethics News* and in *Embryo Experimentation*, edited by Peter Singer *et al.*, published by Cambridge University Press. Dr Miriam Griffin's chapter is a revised version of her article 'Philosophy, Cato, and Roman suicide', in *Greece and Rome* volume XXXIII (April 1986), published by Oxford University Press. Parts of Dr M. Lockwood's chapter have been published in *Bioethics*, issued by Basil Blackwell Ltd. We are grateful to these publishers for permission to reproduce this material here.

1   Introduction: diverse ethics

*K. William M. Fulford, Grant R. Gillett
and Janet M. Soskice*

Books on medical ethics often begin by praising it as a growth industry.
Certainly there is a growing awareness of the importance of medical
ethics, among doctors themselves, among other health care professionals –
nurses, psychologists, social workers – and, most urgently of all, among
those on the receiving end of health care, patients and their families. Some
philosophers, too, readily acknowledge that medical ethics has provided a
timely shot in the arm for their discipline: medicine, Toulmin (1978) says,
has saved the life of philosophy. This book, however, was prompted not
by the growth of interest in medical ethics but, on the contrary, by a
premonition of decline.

The editors of this volume (respectively two physicians and a theologian) were all involved in multi-disciplinary working parties on medical
ethics in Oxford between 1988 and 1990. Here was a good opportunity
for medical ethics, and more particularly philosophical medical ethics,
to make progress: professionals from all sides with the motivation to
combine their experience and skills were tackling well-defined questions in
manageable areas of practice. Here, if anywhere, was a recipe for success.

Yet our experience in these working parties was largely disappointing.
On the safe ground of review there was secure scholarship and sound
opinion. But when it came to new ideas, to pushing the subject forward, in
place of the anticipated fusion of disciplines there was often mutual
incomprehension. To the doctors, conscious of practical imperatives, the
philosophers appeared excessively preoccupied with theory. Philosophical
debate with its tendency to diversity of opinion and approach seemed
hopelessly inconclusive. To the philosophers, on the other hand, the hopes
of the doctors for definite answers, for solutions to the particular
difficulties posed by individual concrete cases, seemed unrealistic. Both
sides, none the less, were conscious of a pressure to perform: reports had
(somehow) to be produced, conclusions (of some kind) had to be
published. But the result was an anodyne, an all too familiar compromise
of a broadly consequentialist kind, unimpeachable yet often unsatisfying.
It was neither sufficiently cognisant of the gritty details faced by pro-

fessionals at the clinical coal-face, nor adequately addressed to the full interest and subtlety of the theoretical issues embodied by these same dilemmas.

One purpose of this book, then, is to reverse this trend towards an unexciting compromise. It seemd to us that the committee mentality, the drift to the mean, was a formula for stagnation in medical–ethical thinking. Rather than merging their distinct identities the two disciplines, we felt, had more to offer each other by maintaining a creative tension.

The collection of essays brought together here reflects this tension. It represents a conscious attempt to pull medical ethics in two directions at once – towards the detail of real clinical experience and, at the same time, towards the diversity of approach that is characteristic of philosophical argument. Encouragingly, among our contributors a pull in the former direction, towards clinical experience, turned out not to be confined to the doctors. The most straightforwardly clinical chapter is by a doctor – Brandt's account of his research on the psychological effects of pre-natal screening for the identification of carriers of the Huntington's disease gene. This study is a paradigm of the value of careful empirical work as a basis for informed medical ethical opinion in a highly contentious area. Similarly, in the concluding chapter, Fulford shows how philosophical analyses of the ethical implications of the concept of illness have been impoverished by a failure to incorporate first-hand clinical data. But an emphasis on 'cases', on the importance of looking at what really happens in the clinical situation, is the theme also of two of our philosophical contributors. Urmson, in particular, argues that medical ethics should be created by doctors from cases upwards rather than by philosophers from theory downwards. Murray, likewise, discusses the importance of the culture-carrying clinical traditions of medicine. Re-introducing the maligned notion of casuistry, he shows how our accumulated professional experience, representing a shared moral tradition, can often illuminate individual cases far more effectively than theoretical arguments constructed in a cultural and historical vacuum.

All this is not to suggest that philosophers are in general indifferent to facts. The importance of close attention to the real world has repeatedly been emphasised by those in the linguistic analytical tradition. In ethics it is no more than a direct corollary of consequentialism, of the view that moral questions should be determined according to the likely outcome of our possible courses of action. In the present volume, Hare defends a version of consequentialism as a tool for determining social policy as distinct from individual ethical decisions. But the message for philosophers, if our experience of working-party ethical discussions is any guide, is that if they are to continue to contribute to the development of medical ethics they must find ways of getting much closer to the primary data of everyday clinical practice.

The corresponding message for doctors is that they must get closer to an understanding of moral philosophy. At one level what is required is plain education. If philosophers have to put in some spade-work to learn medicine, doctors have to put in some spade-work to learn philosophy. But perhaps more fundamental is that doctors should come to see what can and what cannot be expected of philosophy. The philosopher's particular strength is in producing logical and clear arguments (though not always simple ones). In this book Oddie shows how game theory and decision analysis can lead to novel conclusions. And in many other areas of medicine – in classification and diagnosis as well as in ethics – similar formal arguments represent important potential contributions of philosophy to good clinical care. Philosophy can also help us to organise our ideas in more straightforward ways, bringing method and order to the analysis of complex issues. This is one of the merits of the 'principles' approach, though the choice of principles may itself be contentious. In this volume Campbell argues that respect for dependency, rather than autonomy, should be the fundamental principle of medical ethics. But as to answers, as to determinate solutions, off-the-peg ethics for given clinical situations, this is not what philosophy has to offer. Indeed it is characteristic of philosophy that it opens questions up rather than closing them down, that it tests and teases received opinion rather than reinforcing it.

To remind us – philosophers as well as doctors – of this feature of philosophy, is the second main purpose of this book. Closely related to the first, to showing that medicine and philosophy have more to offer each other in their differences than in their similarities, this second purpose is to show that, important as consequentialism is in ethics, there are a large number of other moral philosophical ways to skin the medical ethical cat. Have we forgotten the virtues? May revives this notion here by showing its value to our understanding of the clinical instincts that, in the hasty demands of everyday medical practice, govern our ethical decision making. Have we neglected the historical perspective? Griffin argues that attitudes to death prevalent in Graeco-Roman society, and the philosophical views these reflected, can illumine current ideologies. What of religious ethics? Soskice shows how the beliefs that set such ethics apart, though at risk of generating dogma and inflexibility, may also secure important values of respect for persons, providing a counter-balance to the dehumanising tendency of technological medicine. And what of welfare economics? Crisp examines some of the recent conceptions of welfare which have been employed by health economists active in the political sphere, and finds these conceptions, and the uses to which they have been put, flawed in various ways.

Moral philosophy has of course never existed in isolation from its sister philosophical disciplines, a number of which are represented here. From the current mainstream, Midgley argues against socio-biology as a basis for ethical argument and shows the value to ethics of recent work in the philosophy of science. Attempts to reduce ethics to science, with the object of producing determinate ethical results, are flawed, *inter alia*, by a failure to recognise the extent to which science itself, as a socio-cultural phenomenon, is far from value-free. Despite the shortcomings of science, Lockwood in his chapter on the ethics of abortion, demonstrates the potential of philosophical theories of personal identity which take close account of scientific knowledge about human functioning. Gillett shows how recent accounts of the ways in which we acquire and use concepts in general can lead to a theory of moral reasoning which, in contrast to other attempts to rationalise ethical thinking, is consonant with our most basic moral intuitions.

Diversity then, not uniformity, is the essence of philosophical practice. The selection of philosophical approaches in this book is indeed far from exhaustive. Despite their differences of approach, our contributors are all in the Anglo-American analytical tradition. But hermeneutics has much to offer (Wulff *et al.*, 1986). Similarly, our orientation is essentially 'Western'. But an understanding of other traditions is a prerequisite for sound medical ethics in a multi-cultural society (Tao, 1990). Then again, developmental ethics – concerned with children's understanding of ethical concepts – is providing useful insights (Wolff, 1990). Medical education, too, is beginning to acknowledge the importance of medical ethics. In this area there is still a great deal to be done: what should be taught, by whom, to whom, in what contexts, and by what means? *Practical* medical ethics, after all, is a clinical *skill*, involving communication as much as care; and the acquisition of skills, as a learning process, is known to proceed quite differently from the mere accumulation of facts (Hope and Fulford, forthcoming).

To the doctors on our original Oxford working parties, still conscious of practical imperatives, diversity may seem a recipe for chaos. The idea that philosophical theory should be pulled more firmly towards the facts of clinical life is not, perhaps, contentious. But that it should pull us the other way, towards diversity and divergence? Surely this is incompatible with the clinician's central need for practical decision making, for determinate clinical action?

Yet it is at precisely this point, with the doctor back at the clinical coal-face, that we believe philosophy has most to offer medicine. This is so, first, where there is ethical uncertainty, doubt or disagreement about what ought to be done. It is important to remember that most medicine is not in this way uncertain. Whatever the differences of ethical theory there is often agreement in practice on a wide range of issues (Jonsen, 1986). Even with philosophy at its most iconoclastic, therefore, there is no risk of a generalised ethical paralysis. But where there *are* uncertainties, the contribution of philosophy is not to provide an enervated compromise. It is rather to point up and to make inescapable the true extent of the problems we face. The constraint which medicine provides is indeed the need for decision: *something* has to be done. But philosophy helps us to make better decisions, not by fiat, by by denying us the spurious reassurance of one-sided, confused or otherwise inadequate solutions.

We should seek, then, not the static application of rules but a balanced dynamic of clinical decision making. Philosophy, by fostering diversity of thought, can provide for openness and sensitivity in medical practice and, dare we say, a certain humility! And if this is important where there is uncertainty of ethical view, it is vital where there is consensus. Many of the worst excesses of medical power, the most flagrant misuses of the authority of medicine, have occurred precisely where the confidence necessary for decisive clinical action has been allowed to degenerate into authoritarian dogma. Philosophy should be the gadfly to such medical pretensions.

ACKNOWLEDGEMENTS

The authors are grateful to Dr Roger Crisp and Dr Tony Hope for their helpful comments on an early draft of this chapter.

REFERENCES

Hope, T. and Fulford, K. W. M. (forthcoming) *Medical Education: Patients, Principles and Practice Skills.* R. Gillon (ed.). John Wiley and Sons
Jonsen, A. R. (1986) 'Casuistry and clinical ethics'. *Theoretical Medicine*, 7: 65–74
Tao, J. (1990) 'The Chinese moral ethos and the concept of individual rights'. *Journal of Applied Philosophy*, 7 (2)
Toulmin, S. (1978) 'How medicine saved the life of ethics'. *Perspectives in Biology and Medicine*, 25 (4): 736–50
Wolff, S. (1990) 'Attachment and morality: developmental themes with different values'. *British Journal of Psychiatry*, 156: 266–71
Wulff, H. R., Pedersen, S. A. and Rosenberg, R. (1986) *Philosophy of Medicine, An Introduction.* Oxford: Blackwell Publications

2 Darwinism and ethics

Mary Midgley

Darwinisms

What is Darwinism? The name is often used, not for a scientific theory or group of theories, but for a whole outlook, a system of thought with practical and emotional applications, an ideology. It is seen as a creed, to be attacked or defended, protected or betrayed. What this creed involves varies a lot on different occasions, and can range a long way from Darwin. We need to be much clearer about it. If we do believe – as a fact – the historical story that all existing living species have evolved, over a long time, by natural selection, what does that commit us to? Are there outside commitments, or might it just be an inert fact like many others in science, with no more implications for the rest of life than the periodic number of carbon?

The answer to this will naturally depend, not just on Darwin's actual theory or theories, but on what *other* things we happen to accept already, and what alternatives to them we see as possible. In detail, the problem has changed repeatedly, because the background and the available alternatives are always changing. But right from the start, people have tended to polarize strongly about it because they have thought that crucial issues were involved. There has therefore been a constant temptation to simplify the issues into a struggle of black against white. This has not been only because of religious considerations. As historians have now made very clear, the notion of a simple war between Darwinism and Christianity is quite misleading. Many deeply religious Victorians, such as Charles Kingsley, accepted Darwin's suggestions at once, whereas the scientific establishment treated it with great suspicion. Moreover, anti-Darwinism has flourished vigorously in many quarters which are also hostile to Christianity. Samuel Butler, Bernard Shaw, Arthur Koestler, Fred Hoyle and many other atheists have reprobated fiercely something that they found there. Much of the trouble is not about the position of God at all. It concerns the status of that much more sensitive subject, Man.

Darwin himself foresaw this polarization, which was one reason why he was so slow to publish. He was very tentative in what he said on wider issues, not because he did not realize their importance, but because he did. He took pains to balance his observations and his images, so as to avoid simple and extreme suggestions as much as possible, not just from timidity, but because he saw the vastness of our ignorance on these big subjects. He used a style that was meant to keep many alternative interpretations open until people had had time to bring these difficult matters into focus. Among his successors, however, things have been different. Those who have tried to follow his cautious example have repeatedly been shouted down by more simple-minded champions, confidently issuing narrow and dogmatic manifestos in Darwin's name. We may as well begin our enquiry here by looking at one of these, namely, the colourful story about human agency that crops up from time to time in the works of sociobiologists, more especially in their early ones.

I am not using this point here as part of a general, tribal war or 'sociobiology debate'. In other books, and in other parts of these same books, sociobiologists have done a good job in bringing the idea of 'human nature' back into the field of controversy. But they also convey some very bizarre thought-patterns, among them this extremely peculiar story or myth about how humans act, and they convey them explicitly as part of 'Darwinism'. They display this as something that we ought to accept if we accept the full historical story of evolution. Though the vogue for sociobiology is waning slightly, I think that these mistakes still persist. It is well worth our while to separate them out and consider them on their own merits.

Survival machines and circuitous techniques

The core of this particular myth is the idea that human life is really only a technique or tool used by certain non-human entities – the genes – to achieve aims of their own. As E. O. Wilson (1978) puts it:

(1) Human behaviour – like the deepest capacities for emotional response which drive and guide it – *is* the circuitous technique by which human genetic material has been and will be kept intact. *Morality has no other demonstrable ultimate function.* (Wilson, 1978, p. 167. Emphases mine here and throughout)

It follows, he says, that:

(2) the time has come for ethics to be removed temporarily from the hands of the philosophers and biologicized. (Wilson, 1975, p. 562)

This notion about morality is the central one that I want to discuss, but we need first, as background, some other expressions of the general reductive view about agency:

(3) *We are* survival machines – robot vehicles blindly programmed to preserve the selfish molecules known as genes. This is a *truth* that still fills me with astonishment. (Dawkins, 1976, Introduction, p. x)

(4) The individual organism *is only the vehicle* (of genes), part of an elaborate device to preserve and spread them with the least possible biochemical perturbation . . . The organism *is only* DNA's way of making more DNA. (Wilson, 1975, p. 4)

(Wilson adds that this is a more technical way of putting Samuel Butler's remark that 'the bird is only the egg's way of making more eggs'.)

(5) Thus does ideology bow to its hidden masters, the genes. (Wilson, 1978, p. 4)

(6) Parental love itself *is actually but* an evolutionary strategy whereby genes replicate themselves. (Barash, 1980, p. 3)

What do remarks like these actually mean? In theory they might not be meant to have any practical or emotional consequences for our handling of life. They might just be picturesque ways of stating facts about evolutionary genetics, facts as inert for our lives as the periodic number of carbon. But the extraordinary style in which they are written rules out this interpretation. The metaphors used seem meant in some way to be taken literally; as Dawkins insists, they are 'truths'. And these metaphors are not just violent; they are also so familiar that they unavoidably bring their context with them when we ask how to interpret them. *This is everyday language whose proper and normal use is to describe manipulative fraud.* That stands out clearly if we just change a few words to bring out the ordinary bearing of such words. Thus, the first quotation uses very much the language that we might expect to find used in a Marxist analysis of political constitutions:

(1) Political activity in liberal democracies *is* the circuitous technique by which the power of the ruling class is kept intact. Parliamentary democracy *has no other ultimate function.*

Now it would be very odd (wouldn't it?) to treat this last remark as simply an inert factual report, not meant to have practical or emotional implications. This is an alarm call reporting dangerous deception about matters vitally affecting the common good. It says that devices which we thought were invented and used by one group for public purposes are in fact invented and used by quite a different group for their own private ends. The word 'ultimate' doesn't really mitigate this explosive meaning. It concedes that a little of the official aim may get achieved incidentally on the way, but this concession is so trifling as to be an insult.

With the word *morality* substituted for *parliamentary democracy*, passage (1) cannot fail to convey an exactly parallel message, namely 'morality is just a con', and this is certainly how most readers naturally understand it, whether they rejoice at the news or not. We will come back to what this means later. But to show that this principle of interpretation is not a distorting one, it is worth while first just to use it on some of the metaphors used in the other quotations as well – metaphors that are sprinkled all over these books. Quotation (4) again uses language that is very familiar in a political context, thus:

(4) The press is only the vehicle of capitalist/Marxist propaganda, part of an elaborate device to preserve and spread it with the least possible political perturbation ... The press is only capitalism's/Marxism's way of making more capitalists/Marxists.

Similarly:

(5) Thus does Smith bow to his hidden masters in the Kremlin/CIA.

Or again:

(3) The typical middle-class intellectual is a survival machine, a robot vehicle blindly programmed to preserve the selfish individuals known as millionaires and directors of the multi-national companies. This is a truth which still fills me with astonishment.

Or:

(6) Family affection itself is actually but an emotional strategy whereby capitalism secures a replacement of the work force and thereby perpetuates itself.

Interpretation 1 – Unconscious human motives

Now what actual meaning is the reader expected to attach to all this violent and familiar language in the context of sociobiology? The natural meaning evidently concerns a *deception* – an error which we must penetrate in order to reach a 'truth'. And this has to be self-deception, unless anybody takes the genes to be literally conscious agents doing the deceiving. This is inevitably a view about human motives. It must mean – must it not? – that at some unconscious level our motives are actually quite different from what we profess and believe. What we really want is what our genes have determined us to want – namely, what will best suit *them*. Our pretence of wanting anything else is mere humbug. Barash's title *Sociobiology: The Whisperings Within* strongly supports this interpretation.

In harmony with this approach, sociobiologists, when talking like this, constantly use the anti-humbug language familiar to us from the grand, debunking psychological tradition of Hobbes and Freud – the language that points out how much less respectable our motives are than we would like to imagine. But what they are actually doing is totally different. People like Hobbes and Freud are contrasting one human motive with another. They have to bring concrete, detailed evidence from within human life to support these diagnoses, and where that evidence is not good enough, we don't accept their reductive findings.

The sociobiologists, however, don't bring that kind of evidence at all – indeed, they often explain that they are not even talking about particular motives, but about something that is necessarily true of all motives. They argue entirely *a priori*, from general principles. The contrast they draw is not between any two human motives, but between a human motive and something that is not a motive at all but a general cause of the existence of motives – namely, the influence of genes. *These things are not alternatives and establishing the one can do nothing to exclude the other.* They are different kinds of explanation, answering different questions. Just so, one might 'explain' the Koh-i-noor on the one hand by describing the general constitution of diamonds from carbon, and on the other by its individual history – telling how diamonds have come to be highly valued and how this particular one came to be a trophy of Empire. There is no inference between the two stories and no possible ground for reductive nothing-buttery.

Interpretation 2 – The 'motives' of genes

Are we missing something here? Is there actually some reason why motives which have genes among their causes always will be of a crude, egoistic kind, because only these motives could serve the survival of genes? Readers of these books certainly do get that impression, the crude motive involved being taken to be 'selfishness' in the ordinary sense of that word. But the authors, on their good days, officially reject this interpretation, and, since the early books quoted here, Dawkins and Wilson at least have steadily drawn away from endorsing it. Officially, sociobiological theory supposes that it is *genes*, not individuals, that are 'selfish'. In order for the genes to be maximally spread, it must often happen that the individual must be sacrificed.

Indeed, *sociobiology arose originally as a way of explaining the given fact of altruism*, an attempt to make intelligible the finding that behaviour, both in plants and animals, was not at all consistently individualistic and self-interested. Yet, because the egoistic habit of thinking was so in-grained, this fact was colourfully expressed by saying that self-interest belonged to the genes rather than to the individuals. This made it almost impossible for the authors to remain clear about what they were doing.

Elements of the regular Hobbesian propaganda for egoism constantly flowed from their pens, and brought their familiar, personal context along with them. For instance:

(7) Compassion is selective and often self-serving; ... it conforms to the best interests of self, family and allies of the moment. (Wilson, 1978, pp. 154–5)

(8) Like successful Chicago gangsters, our genes have survived, in some cases for millions of years, in a highly competitive world. This entitles us to expect certain qualities in our genes. I shall argue that a predominant quality to be expected in a successful gene is ruthless selfishness ... If you wish, as I do, to build a society in which individuals co-operate generously towards a common good, you can expect little help from biological nature. Let us try to *teach* generosity and altruism, because *we are born selfish.* (Dawkins, 1976, p. 2)

(9) We will analyse parental behaviours, the underlying selfishness of our behaviour towards others, even our own children. (Barash, 1980, p. 3)

Astonishingly, both these last two pronouncements occur in the opening pages of books, before there has been any suggestion at all of redefining the term 'selfishness'.

(10) The evolution of society fits the Darwinian paradigm in its most individualistic form. The economy of nature is competitive from beginning to end ... No hint of genuine charity ameliorates our vision of society, once sentimentalism has been laid aside. What passes for cooperation turns out to be a mixture of opportunism and exploitation. The impulses that lead one animal to sacrifice himself for another turn out to have their ultimate rationale in gaining advantage over a third ... Where he has no alternative, he submits to the yoke of servitude. Yet, given a full chance to act in his own interest, nothing but expediency will restrain him from brutalizing, from maiming, from murdering – his brother, his mate, his parent or his child. Scratch an 'altruist' and watch a 'hypocrite' bleed. (M. T. Ghiselin, 1974, p. 147)

All this bizarre rhetoric is quite contrary to the basic position of sociobiology, which admits the frequent occurrence of individual altruism and claims only that behaviour must be such that it has promoted the survival of existing genes.

What are evolutionary functions?

With this remarkable confusion about selfishness out of the way, let us go back to the somewhat mysterious passage from which we started. What does it mean to say that 'morality has no other demonstrable ultimate function' except to be part of the 'circuitous technique by which human genetic material has been and will be kept intact? In what sense is this a function, and an ultimate function? Words like 'function' are most easily intelligible when used in relation to the purposes of conscious beings, as with tools and houses. But of course the parts of living beings can also have functions even where no conscious purpose is present to guide them, as with plants. Following Aristotle, we call these parts *organs*, which is simply the Greek word for tools. Here the assumed purpose is provided by the possible benefits of the whole organism, including its survival. More widely still, these beings can also have other characteristics which do not promote their own survival, but which do promote the survival of their kin, and so of their genes and of their species. Many social tendencies are of this kind, and this seems to be the kind of function which is being allotted to morality here. It makes sense, then, to call it an evolutionary function.

But if we say that morality has this function, we are not saying much about it. For the very same thing can be said, with equal confidence or equal hesitation, about all pervasive human social tendencies and the arrangements to which they give rise. Exactly this same function which is attributed to morality must then also be attributed to music, to speech, to laughter and joking, to revenge, to dancing and poetry, to gambling, to arguing and abstract enquiry, to friendship and love and many more. All these are tendencies which seem built into human nature everywhere, and which therefore – as I would entirely agree with the sociobiologists – probably are innate, and probably had some use in forming the social way of life by which our species has survived and prospered.

This tells us nothing at all about the *function* of each of them in the ordinary sense in which we might ask about it. Our question then would surely be: just what distinctive part did each of these various elements in life play, and what part can they now play, in the life of various human societies? No doubt, from the remote, theoretical point of view of someone studying comparative evolution, the general idea that these things must all have brought some kind of advantage can sometimes be important. But from the inside – from the angle of a human being trying to understand human life – it is the *difference* between these various advantages that usually matters.

If we ask about the function of morality, we will be asking just what it does for people, what difference it makes in their lives, why they need it, and how they would get on without it – if indeed life without it would be possible at all. There is no obvious way in which this question could be called less 'ultimate' than the one about evolutionary effects. It is certainly not less serious. They are simply different questions, arising out of different enquiries.

It is possible, indeed, that 'ultimate' here isn't meant to mean serious or important, but simply long-term, indicating that this is the function most likely to remain constant through all changes over a very long period of time. That may be true in a rather empty and peculiar sense, perhaps in the same sense, indeed, in which the ultimate function of everything in the physical universe might be said to be 'to bring about universal entropy'. But it gives this question-and-answer no kind of priority over the other. The inward, more practically urgent question is the one from the internal point of view, on which Darwin himself made some good suggestions. Since this is also the question likely to occur to most readers on hearing talk of 'the ultimate function of morality', answering it, as Wilson appears to, with the answer belonging to a quite different and much remoter question is seriously misleading. People naturally take 'ultimate' to mean 'most important'. Wilson's answer suggests that the functions we might suppose morality to have – functions such as harmonizing human life and clearing it of its more horrible elements – are somehow unreal, superficial, perhaps plain delusory. Morality, it now seems, does not really do this work; its 'only ultimate function' is to preserve and spread human genes. Readers will naturally infer that they have been had and that, if they wish to be smart, they should pay less regard to morality for the future. That is almost certainly not Wilson's intention, but it is the natural conclusion to draw from his words.

Reductive habits and the position of animals

This example brings us back to our earlier question of what bothers people so much about what is broadly called 'Darwinism'. The thing that does bother them is surely a diffused impression of habitual reductiveness – of a temper always ready to bundle large and important things away under small and inadequate headings and dismiss them without proper attention. Because the whole topic of evolution is so large, there are many places where this can happen, and it is important to deal with each on its merits. It often then emerges that the reductiveness isn't present in a proper, careful statement of what is happening, but that it lurks in the background unrecognized by its owners, and subtly distorts the forms of statement that theorists use.

This case of the 'function of morality' is surely of that kind. It is one where a belief in natural selection as a causal factor is wrongly thought to *compete* with something of value – namely, in this case, recognition of our immense psychological complexity and of its bearing on this subtle function. The fact that our emotional constitution has evolved by natural selection doesn't imply at all that it is crude, simple and egoistic. Many of the products of natural selection are incredibly complex – think of a termite's nest or a colonial jellyfish – and the interworking pressures of social life seem calculated to produce something at least as intricate as any of these. In fact they have produced a rich variety of non-egoistic behaviour among social animals, and produced it long before human beings came on the scene.

This last fact is important, because one reason why people tend to think that an evolutionary history must degrade and simplify our motivation has of course been that they already had a very misleading, reductive impression about the natures of the social animals from whom we have evolved. It has been a most important part of Darwinian work to correct just that misleading impression. The traditional idea of animals as crassly insensitive and simple, or as automata, or sometimes as mere embodiments of vice, is quite unrealistic, simply a projection of our own fantasies tailored to justify our exploitative practices towards them.

The truth about these animals' complex natures is far more fascinating, and its gradual revelation in this century by patient and systematic ethologists, such as Jane Goodall, has been one of the humanistic, as well as one of the scientific triumphs of our time. That is to say, it has been a great contribution to our understanding of our own lives, as well as to our understanding of the world around us. If we do not grasp our links with that world, we cannot properly understand ourselves. And here Darwinism has been far from reductive – indeed it has been admirably expansive, if that is the proper word for the contrast. Darwin himself was filled with a deep reverence for the world he studied, with the kind of awe and wonder that earlier philosophers such as Aristotle and Spinoza had described in religious terms as a response to its divinity. This spirit corrects the destructive element of contempt and hatred for the natural world which has sometimes been present in Christianity, and which has if anything been intensified in our culture by secular developments during the Enlightenment and the Industrial Revolution. Human arrogance and claustrophobic obsession with local projects need this corrective. Once we apply it, our eyes are no longer closed to the marvellous subtlety of natural systems, and we no longer feel any compulsion to pretend that the animals that surround us are simple machines, or systems of stimulus-response reflexes, or to enclose them in any other unrealistic distancing and alienating conceptual scheme.

The idea that kinship with these animals is necessarily degrading should then evaporate. We begin to see, too, that such a kinship does not call on us to deny the complexity or the uniqueness of human life. We are indeed unique, as also are elephants, bees, gorillas and every other highly social life-form. Each has its own peculiar features. Each would have been unimaginable had we only had the others to conjecture it from. There is no such thing as a standard animal. There exists no boring, basic mechanical model to which we need feel that we are being reduced. One thing that a more respectful attitude to the physical world does for us is to give us a sense of perspective about the immense range of this variation, an awareness of the wide conceptual space in which this range of creatures is deployed. Once we grasp this vastness, we no longer need to feel the horror of imprisonment in too narrow a category – a claustrophobic horror which has certainly formed a great part of the objection people have felt to being classed as 'animals'.

Reverence for life

This liberating sense of reverence for the vast kingdom of nature can do away with the reductive impression that many people get from the theory of evolution. By ceasing to be so reductive about the natural world itself, we can begin to feel that to be at home in it, and to belong to it, is not an affront to human dignity, but is our proper and honourable position. Is this reverent attitude, however, itself a part of 'Darwinism'?

It is not, of course, an unfailing consequence of the belief that there has been an evolutionary process. Plenty of contemporary biologists accept that belief but entirely lack the reverence. Unimaginative people, fully occupied with their test-tubes and their computers, do not need reverence to make them work on a particular subject-matter. Money or ambition will do instead. Very many *good* biologists, however, do have this reverence, and connect it explicitly with the evolutionary story. Many of them have said, too, that this reverence is essential equipment for doing really good biology. Historically, it is a motive that has been very influential, not only in Darwin himself, but in most of the great naturalists of the past who have contributed to uncovering this remarkable story. Reverence of this kind furnishes a suitably powerful motive to direct the mass of hard thinking, the wide yet disciplined speculations that have been necessary if they were to do this work on a scale appropriate to the subject-matter.

In any case, whether or not it might have been possible for other attitudes to lead to the discovery of evolution, if Darwin's name is to be attached to a general attitude, and not just a factual theory, it seems important that that attitude should be his and not that of other people who have since hijacked his bandwagon. That spirit is above all a tentative and reverent one. When, therefore, we find his name confidently invoked in support of extreme ideologies such as that of Ghiselin in quotation (10), our reply should be, not just to debunk the ideology, but also to say 'leave Darwin alone'.

Conclusion – do we really believe Darwin's story?

I have tried, in this article, to break up the cluster of diverse views currently suggested by the term 'Darwinism' so as to make it easier for people to identify what they want to attack and defend, what they mind and what they don't in that loose but highly charged cluster. My first hope is indeed that readers can carry this process further – that they will now find it easier to resist being bulldozed into accepting or rejecting something simply by the claim that it is an integral part of Darwinism. Next, I have concentrated on certain particular objectionable and (to my mind) dangerous notions – very anti-Darwinian notions – which are today often treated as part of the cluster. My reason for making this attack is not mere destructiveness, but, first, that these notions are troublesome in themselves, and second, that removing them may make it easier to see what should actually be the metaphysical shape of evolutionary thinking. I have pursued this rather indirect, negative method instead of instantly trying to describe that shape, because I think in general that removing gross and vivid errors is often necessary before one can see the outlines of what is left behind well enough to deal with its larger problems.

I take those larger problems, however, very seriously. As many people have pointed out, we still lack a clear-headed way of imagining the world, and ourselves in it, which really accepts the historical story to which our biology and geology officially commit us. Countless odd contemporary thought-movements, ranging from Creationism to strange, neo-Lamarckian prophecies of a future scientific progress to disincarnated immortality and omnipotence, show how hard many of us still find it to accommodate ourselves to being part of the natural world. I think the best thing I can do here is to end by briefly summarizing Darwin's own response to this question about the function of morality. I find it an exceptionally helpful attempt to make intelligible what is surely the crux of this imaginative problem about evolution – how we can, without degradation, suppose the more admirable features of human life to have arisen out of something that was non-human.

What, then, *is* the function of morality? Eighteenth-century rationalism gave a very clear answer, saying that primitive men, being intelligent and prudent egoists, had seen that they would be safer if they all made a social contract not to injure each other. It thus set up moral rules on the ground of enlightened self-interest. Darwin, however, was in a position to point out that that simple answer could not possibly be right, because there had never been any such primitive men occupying that primal position. Instead, there had been social mammals who, long before humanity ever existed, had begun to love and help those around them on the ground, not of prudence, but of natural affection. Human beings were descended from these mammals, and quite evidently were not inferior to them in these natural affections. Our primate ancestors therefore could not possibly have had either the powers of prudent calculation or the coldly solitary emotional constitution demanded by the social contract myth. They did not wait to acquire them; they became deeply social before ever they expanded their cerebral cortices.

That does not mean that the contract myth is useless. It has important uses in political situations, where we want to stress that certain particular social arrangements are optional. But to suggest that consideration for those around us has ever been optional in this way – that there was a time, or could ever be a situation, where people might decide just to live as self-contained egoists – is biological nonsense. The long dependency of our children alone is enough to explode it. 'Immoralism', if taken to mean that kind of consistent egoism or moral solipsism, is not a conceivable option for human beings.

As Darwin pointed out, social affections alone do not amount to a morality. But how about social affections in combination with an increased intelligence? As the cortex did expand, and wider thinking became possible, early people could become aware of how unevenly their affections were working. Improving memory, along with increased power of thinking about the future, would bring back past actions for repeated scrutiny, so that they – unlike any of their ancestors – would become capable of being haunted by what they had done, and of wanting to do differently henceforward. Remorse and regret, says Darwin, would surely become urgent, and the natural way to control remorse and regret would be to work out policies for the future that would stop them recurring. (See *The Descent of Man* volume I, part i chapter 5, 'On the development of the intellectual and moral faculties', especially p. 91.)

Thus rules would begin to be formed – not all at once (as the contract model may suggest) but gradually, through a process involving continual developments both in thought and feeling, a process which is open-ended and is still going on today. That is why this is not a reductive account. Darwin does *not* say 'the function of morality is simply to defuse remorse' or the like. He knows that the functions we find for it will develop as we ourselves develop. In the great flexibility of human cultures, we can gradually identify many different ideals and grow remorseful about many different things. But what he does succeed in doing is showing how we could start the process from our mammalian base, without requiring the special divine intervention which Alfred Wallace thought must have been needed to launch humanity. To put the point in more timeless, less historical terms – Darwin shows how vital our emotional constitution is to all that we most admire, he enables us to accept and celebrate duly this emotional constitution which is so close to that of the other social animals, instead of insisting that everything we value is the work of that overstrained and hypertrophied cerebral cortex. He leaves us at home with our own nature and on the earth. And if 'Darwinism' has to be regarded as a creed, that is the message in it which I would most want us to accept.

REFERENCES

For any readers interested in the ramifications of my own position – I have discussed the phenomenon of sociobiology more fully in my *Beast and Man* (Methuen, 1978), especially in its introduction, and have tried to do fuller justice to Darwin's moral views in *Wickedness a Philosophical Essay* (Routledge, 1984) chapter 9, 'Evil in evolution'. I have also considered the role of non-Darwinian fantasies about escalator-type evolution in *Evolution as a Religion* (Methuen, 1985) and in *Science of Salvation* (Routledge, 1992).

Barash, David (1980) *Sociobiology: The Whisperings Within*. London: Souvenir Press

Darwin, Charles (1981) *The Descent of Man*. Reprint of the first edition (1871). Princeton University Press

Dawkins, Richard (1976) *The Selfish Gene*. Oxford University Press

Ghiselin, M. T. (1974) *The Economy of Nature and the Evolution of Sex*. Berkeley, CA: University of California Press

Wilson, E. O. (1975) *Sociobiology: The New Synthesis*. Boston, MA: Harvard University Press

(1978) *On Human Nature*. Boston, MA: Harvard University Press

3   Creation and relation

Janet Martin Soskice

Medical ethics committees almost inevitably have theologians amongst their members, something of a curiosity in a society like ours which, we are told, is largely indifferent to religious matters. Why not rely on the philosophers alone? Why is it that theologians who work in the area of medical ethics are rung up with regularity by media folk who want a religious point of view? Is it simply a moral nostalgia at work, or yet a hunt for a reactionary opinion to contrast with up-to-date views? I think not. Rather there seems an inkling, even amongst those who are not themselves of a religious disposition, that these old ways and even the old myths may have something still to tell us about human well-being and our being in the world.

From the theologian's point of view, membership of a medical ethics working party can be a frustrating experience, not through lack of things to say or people who are willing to listen, but because moral judgements in any complex religion are based on a network of metaphysical and religious beliefs. In some senses, for instance, to understand the Christian view of the dignity of human life you have to go back to the Jewish and Christian myths of creation and this, in the context of a busy working party, there is rarely time to do.

In this chapter I try to embed some of the distinctive theological beliefs about the dignity of the human person in a wider theology of creation and relation, with some attendant discussion along the way of the manner in which contemporary theology and modern science relate one with another, and the way both might contribute not only to our evaluations of what is appropriate behaviour with regard to other human beings, but with what should be our attitude to the rest of the created order as well. From a religious point of view these things cannot ultimately be separated from one another.

The very title of the book of Genesis means 'origins', but origins of what? Recent works on creation and theology have dealt extensively, sometimes almost exclusively, with questions about the origins of the physical universe and its life forms. The scientists deferred to have been astrophysicists, and the covers of the books bear pictures of swirling galaxies. For a whole generation of doctrinal theologians and philosophers of religion (my generation) this is what theology of creation meant – talk of big bangs and 'fine tuning' of the physical variables which make life possible. Certainly Genesis is concerned with the creation of the physical order but it is also concerned with the creation of the people, Israel, too, with order and right relation. In its first chapters we are given a schematic outline of the relation of the human being to God, the relation of man to woman, of human beings to plants and animals and to each other. Throughout Christian history these chapters of Genesis have been plundered to provide pictures of the ideal humanity, the ideal marriage, even the ideal State. The concerns of Genesis then are both wider and narrower, different from, those of the modern physical and biological scientist.

One common feature of this ancient religious text and modern science, however, is a concern with ultimate origins. Some of the earliest examples of biblical commentary we have are the Hexaemera, so called because they gave an account of the first six days of Creation. One of their objects was to insist that all that is was created freely by God. In posing their challenges to pagan creation narratives they sought to do so in ways compatible with the received scientific knowledge of their own day, a feature of the Hexaemera which impressed the nineteenth-century philosopher of science, Pierre Duhem. We can imagine that St Augustine, too, would have approved, for he thought that Christians made themselves ridiculous when they talked 'utter nonsense' about scientific matters while claiming to speak in accordance with Scripture. This makes Christian writers into laughing-stocks, he said, and does great harm, for when non-Christians hear a Christian making bizarre claims about the physical world and justifying them by appeal to Scripture, 'how are they to believe the same writings on the resurrection of the dead in the hope of eternal life in the kingdom of heaven?'. According to Augustine, in a text much admired and appealed to by Galileo, 'whatever the [scientists] themselves can demonstrate by true proofs about the nature of things, we can show not to be contrary to our scriptures'.[1]

This conciliatory attitude to natural science strikes us as modern on Augustine's part, for we have entered in recent decades another period of amiable relations between science and religion. In one way or another theology has come to terms with the challenges our great-grandparents faced in Darwinism – no longer do we find ourselves in the place of Ruskin whose faith wavered with each tap of the geologist's hammer. Indeed in recent decades some theologians have regarded science not as an enemy but as an ally and have called attention to strategies of scientific theory-construction and model-building in defence of their own strategies of theory-construction and model-building. As modern science has become more eloquent about its own limitations and the difficulty and tentativeness of any truth-claims, theologians have been emboldened to make comparisons with their own tasks.[2] Advances in cosmology and evolutionary biology have even encouraged the more reckless among the philosophers of religion in the ever-elusive hope that one day science will prove that God exists. A number of conferences have taken place on epistemology, metaphysics, theology and astrophysics.

For those of us interested in science and religion this is all gratifying but also somewhat alarming. Why do our collections of essays always have that swirling galaxy on the cover, or a piece of electron-microscopical photography, and never a baby's foot or a woman drawing water at a well, or – to use a biblical image of creation – a rainbow? As our essays on creation become ever more dense and theoretical there is a danger that they become ever more remote not only from what (if anything) the biblical books say about such things, but from what the Christian tradition ever wanted to say. Biblical scholars who somehow managed to 'gate-crash' science and religion symposia are often appalled at what passes for the Christian theology of creation. Is there not a danger that we are engaged in an elaborate parlour game which, however fascinating, is one which very few indeed will ever be able to play? Is this just a new scholasticism which, despite real merits, is as destined as its late-medieval predecessor for obsolescence?

As a contributor to some of these discussions I want to say, 'No'. These discussions are important in an overall Christian apologetic, and their obscurity to the non-professional is neither here nor there. (Few lay people understand modern astrophysics but they would understand well enough if someone claimed that modern astrophysics had decisively demonstrated that God could not exist.) But I wish to raise the spectre of the parlour game to highlight a kind of schizophrenia in the science and religion dialogue at present. For while doubt may be cast on the immediate impact of the lofty, metaphysical discussions currently taking place between scientists and theologians, there is no room to doubt the immediate impact science and scientific practice are having on all our everyday lives. One can scarcely even begin to list the areas of moral concern on which scientific theory and practice have some bearing: computer fraud, the disposal of industrial waste, *in vitro* fertilization, the development and cost of armaments, the allocation of medical resources, the generation and limitation of world famine, AIDS, pollution, ante-natal diagnosis of genetic diseases. Wherever we turn we see possibilities, but also dangers. Even well-intentioned efforts may have unfortunate, even disastrous side effects. The hardy and disease-resistant crops that we hope will transform the lives of people in poor countries may need expensive fertilizers which only the rich can buy. Thus the introduction of the crops may serve to concentrate land and wealth in the hands of those already landed and wealthy, rather than aid the subsistence farmer who was originally supposed to benefit. These moral issues may not, as with positivist challenges of an earlier era, pose a threat to Christian belief *per se*, but they do represent a challenge to which Christianity, if it is to continue in its vision, must rise.

These issues are not issues for the Christians alone – they are all citizens' problems, and indeed all nations' problems, since many extend beyond the scope of a personal ethics. I may independently decide when pregnant not to take the alpha-fetoprotein tests which may indicate neurological disorders, but I cannot decide as an individual how to dispose of nuclear waste. However, even if these are not exclusively Christian problems, none the less may we not hope for some guidance from our religious beliefs as we move cautiously forward?

This is the point at which the schizophrenia in science and religion bites. After some time doing research in the philosophy of religion and philosophy of science I was a member of a working party in medical ethics. This group, composed in the main of medical doctors, philosophers and theologians, was discussing 'Quality of Life in Medical Decision-Making'. The contrast with my former involvement with science and religion was sharp. Whereas the science and religion debate at the 'swirling galaxies' level was fizzing with ideas and happy meetings of mind, one felt in the area of medical ethics that one was entering a conceptual wasteland, one where theological contribution was both peripheral and impoverished. Who was to blame? Not the scientists. They were coming simply with problems, one of the biggest of which was, 'On what basis do I make judgements about or between human lives?'. One doctor said, 'I can't tell you exactly when a patient has died: I can tell you when her heart stops beating, or when she stops breathing independently, or when there's no pulse or no brain activity, but to say exactly when she has died – that's no longer a medical judgement'. The scientific contribution was, one could say, morally neutral. Blame, if there is blame, must be laid at the doors of the moral theologians (amongst whom for these purposes I place myself) for the signal failure to match with theologically compelling arguments the self-confident and increasingly aggressive views of moral atheism.

In such circumstances the cry goes up for the 'Christian opinion' – that is why theologians are asked on to medical ethics working parties in the first place. But 'Christian opinion' does not amount to theological argument; for example, a Roman Catholic theologian might be expected to express the 'opinion' that experimenting on embryos is wrong, but with no scope or opportunity to explain on what rational basis, in the light of their religious beliefs, Catholics might hold such a conviction. Rather this is seen as just one opinion thrown in by an interest group.

If the theologian should defend the opinion, she or he would be expected to do so on what was assumed to be the neutral ground of secular moral philosophy. From there these debates always proceed in a predictable way. The same questions perennially occur and perennially fail to be resolved: When does life begin? Is the embryo a 'person'? What weight should be given to potential?, etc., with scarcely a glance at what bearing Christian doctrine might have on such matters.

In such circumstances the theologian usually colludes in playing on ground which, far from being neutral, is home ground to secular moral philosophy and a wasteland for moral theology. No wonder, then, the impoverishment almost to the point of extinction of a distinctive theological voice. All the Christian can do in such circumstances is to offer his 'opinion' in a louder voice, but since there is no real conversation, no meeting of minds, the voice is unlikely to be heard.

Even in the Christian press today the discussion of controversial moral issues often takes the form of raised voices and embattled opinions, with little reference to the theological and biblical roots which gave rise to and make sense of these views. This shouting technique is unlikely to persuade non-Christians who do not share one's views, but even worse, it is increasingly unlikely to convince rank-and-file believers either, especially when the milieu in which they (for the most part) move is one increasingly alienated from Christian moral assumptions.

An example which to me demonstrates the gap opening up between Christian and agnostic moral assumptions comes from Peter Singer and Helga Kuhse's book, *Should the Baby Live?*, a book which deals with the problems of handicapped infants and the morality of infanticide. Singer and Kuhse go far beyond simply ignoring Christian views; they attack Christianity as the dominating and restrictive ideology which has, for so many centuries, curtailed human freedoms in the West. For more than 1500 years, they state, Christianity has dominated Western moral thought. Those who rejected it were persecuted. 'During this long era of totalitarian enforcement, Christian moral views gained an almost unshakeable grip on our moral thinking.'[3] We must detach ourselves from them if we are to address the moral issue of severely handicapped infants. In particular we must detach ourselves from the idea that human life has a special sanctity, a belief which may be defensible within certain religions but which cannot carry conviction in a pluralist state.

Let me remind you that Singer and Kuhse's argument is not directed towards abortion but infanticide – the killing of newborns who might otherwise live. If one includes in the definition of 'human' such indicators as self-awareness, self-control, sense of future and past, then Kuhse and Singer are content. But simply to be a member of the species *homo sapiens* is not enough to make a being 'human' in the sense necessary for life to be preserved. Many disabled babies will never be 'human' in this more rigorous sense. Why, their argument continues, should being a *homo sapiens* be so overridingly important? Is not this just species-ism, and much analogous to a racism wherein killing a black is less morally significant than killing a white? Species, like race and sex, Singer and Kuhse argue, is a morally irrelevant distinction.

They blame Christianity for the dominance in our culture of this morally irrelevant distinction, and in particular the doctrine that man (*sic*) is made in the image of God, licensed to kill other creatures but not his or her own kind. But according to Singer and Kuhse, 'an inquiring sceptic would wonder why an anencephalic infant (one born with little or no brain) more closely resembles God than, say, a pig.' Their conclusion is that 'to allow infanticide before the onset of self-awareness ... cannot threaten anyone who is in a position to worry about it'.[4]

One should not dismiss their argument summarily. Singer's earlier book, *Animal Liberation*, was a considerable success amongst anti-species-ists, some of whom – one imagines – had little idea that advancing the cause of animals could have such radical implications for the claims of disabled human babies. But what is most interesting is that Singer and Kuhse place the essence of the debate in theology. While Christian ethics has been at pains to play on the grounds of secular philosophy, here we find two secular writers throwing the ball firmly into the theological court.

I would like now to sketch the beginning of a response to the accusation that the 'the traditional principle of the sanctity of human life is the outcome of some seventeen centuries of Christian domination of Western thought and cannot rationally be defended',[5] and this brings us back to the theology of creation, a topic to which those of us interested in the debate between science and religion must now look with some urgency.

The theologies of creation which can be traced in the Old and New Testaments are not primarily interested in cosmology, and throughout Christian history, although theologians have occasionally pondered such questions as whether the universe had a beginning in time or whether it did not, these were never the central theological questions. Thomas Aquinas could suppose either possibility to be compatible with the Christian doctrine that God is creator, although he believed, as a matter of fact, that the universe did have a beginning.

The biblical discussions of creation seem concerned not so much with where the world came from as with *who* it came from, not so much with what kind of creation it was in the first place as with what kind of creation it was and is *now*.[6] Creation in the Old Testament is, above all, order and it comes from God, exclusively from God. God is sovereign in creation and does not tinker with pre-existing matter like some demiurge. In Genesis God creates the universe from nothing and effortlessly. God pushes back the waters and separates light from dark. Creation is the triumph of order over chaos, and because creation is order it is law-abiding and, according to the Genesis story, it is initially both peaceable and just.

Later theologies posited that God, as creator of all that is, is both mysteriously Other (for God is not a creature) and also totally intimate to everything. God as both Otherness and Intimacy is, as Martin Buber insists, the 'You that in accordance with its nature cannot become an it'.[7] God, too, is mystery – the mystery by which we humans and all the rest of the created order are held in being. Christians believe that in Jesus of Nazareth the Word became flesh but not, as Karl Barth ceaselessly pointed out, that the God who is mystery becomes unmysterious in Jesus Christ. If we don't see Jesus Christ as mystery we see not God incarnate but a great man.

Human beings have a privileged role to play in God's creative love because, according to this story, they are made in the image of God. This, of course, is anthropocentrism, but not necessarily in a hostile form. One can distinguish two versions of Christian anthropocentrism, both of which have had their advocates. In what we might call 'divine hamster cage' anthropocentrism, God is the hamster owner and we are the hamsters. God creates the world as a kind of vivarium for human beings. The rest of the created order is our lettuce leaves and clean sawdust, completely at our disposal – quite literally, the world is our 'environment'. (This by the way is a very good reason for never speaking about 'The Environment' and talking instead of 'Creation'.) In what we might call 'divine servant' or 'divine regent' anthropocentrism, on the other hand, human beings are integrally part of the whole of the created order but they have a privileged responsibility within it; rights are attended by responsibility. Women and men are made 'in the image of God' not to ravage God's creation but to attend to it, both by caring for it and by praising it.

Whatever else it may mean to say the human person is in the image of God, it must mean, as Eastern Orthodoxy has insisted, that the human person, like the Deity, is in some sense a mystery. It is this doctrine of 'the person in the image of God' which, for the Church Fathers, keeps the human being from 'being finally dissected by reason'.[8] When we meet another person, however poor, lowly, diseased or dumb, we stand before something which holds the divine – we stand before someone who is mystery and must be reverenced as such, someone who, like Buber's God, is a 'You that in accordance with its nature cannot become an it'. Of course we can, and do, treat other people like 'its', as mere objects, but always to the loss of our own humanity. We do this in pornography, in harmful experiments on unwitting human victims, in indiscriminate killing in war. Ironically we can treat our neighbours as so many 'its' precisely in our eagerness to understand how they work. We are often, as Andrew Louth has said, bewildered by mysteries that remain mysterious even when disclosed. But, he continues:

if in our encounter with others we come to control and dominate them, and are not content to allow them their freedom in which they ultimately escape our understanding and control, then we have ceased to treat them as persons. In dominating them we depersonalize them, and ourselves. As Simone Weil put it, might's 'power to transform a man into a thing is double and it cuts both ways'; it petrifies differently but equally the souls of those who suffer it, and of those who wield it.[9]

God is mystery, and woman and man in God's image are mystery. The death of God will not, as Nietzsche thought, result in the glorification of man, but rather will take from women and men any claim they may have to be reverenced as participating in the divine economy. Without God and without the sanctity of the person made in the image of God, women and men will become not gods but mere objects to manipulate in a world of manipulable objects; and thus Singer and Kuhse.

It is both salutary and confusing that the Genesis story should tell us that it is this same creature, made in the image of God, through whom sin and violence disrupt the created order. Adam and Eve disobey God, Cain slays Abel. In the story violence spreads from the human realm to that of the animals. In the garden the animals live peaceably with Adam and Eve and with each other. After the Flood, we are told, they dread them. The point of these stories is that sin keeps us not only from right relation to other people but from right relation to the whole created order. But the earth and all its life are, after all, destroyed in the Flood, for the God who creates is also the God who saves – a theme strong in both Testaments. The God who saves Noah and the animals can save his people Israel, and – so Christians assert – save humanity in Christ. A God who creates can save. 'Our help is in the name of the Lord', says the Psalmist, 'who made heaven and earth' (Ps. 124.8).

The prophet Isaiah prayed for a just king who, as God's regent over creation, would be a saviour to his people, who would bring order and banish chaos. This king would judge the poor with justice and strike down the ruthless; and then, when there was justice, there would be peace. Then, only then, says Isaiah, lapsing into visionary language, 'The wolf shall dwell with the lamb . . . and the calf and the lion and the fatling together, and a little child shall lead them' (Isa. 11.6–7). This is a vision of Paradise, the New Creation, the Kingdom of God. We should not let the visionary nature of Isaiah's language distract us from the reality of the call. Robert Murray puts it thus:

> The Bible teaches us that neither sin nor salvation are affairs merely between us humans and God; sin entails alienation from our nature which relates us to God's other creatures, while salvation entails our re-integration in a vaster order and harmony which embraces the whole cosmos.[10]

Reverence for and right relation with God entail reverence for and right relation with other people who are made in the image of God, and further they involve right relation with the rest of the created order. The ethical imperative in this vision for the personal extends into the social and finally into the natural and cosmological.

On such a broad canvas religious writers from the biblical times onwards have painted a picture of God's creative and redeeming love. We might, I believe, in our discussions of the moral issues in science and religion, paint on a similarly broad canvas at least part of the time: Whatever we come up with must have regard, as St Augustine would have insisted, for the best science and for what we know of ourselves as creatures – of our biology, our psychology, our natural genesis. Yet we remain mysterious, for we stand in an odd position – fragments of the universe which are conscious of themselves as precisely that. The pop-singer, Joni Mitchell, put it this way in a song written over twenty years ago:

> We are stardust. Million-year-old carbon.
> We are golden. Caught in the devil's bargain
> And we've got to get ourselves back to the garden.[11]

She is basically right. Science agrees with Scripture in this – we are dust, million-year-old carbon. But we are dust that has come to know itself as dust, to know that dust can do right and commit wrongs. Let us start from there.

NOTES

1 Augustine, *The Literal Meaning of Genesis (De Genesi ad litteram)*. Trans. J. H. Taylor (1982) New York: Newman Press, I, xix, 39; V, iii, 3.
2 See Soskice (1985) *Metaphor and Religious Language*. Oxford University Press for a more detailed account.
3 Helga Kuhse and Peter Singer (1985) *Should the Baby Live?: The Problem of Handicapped Infants*. Oxford University Press, p. 117.

4 *Ibid.*, pp. 124 and 138.

5 *Ibid.*, p. 125.

6 It would be misleading, of course, to say that the Old and/or New Testaments have one unified 'theology of creation'. The reader must forgive me if I speak rather loosely here. My remarks however are based on recent work on creation themes in the biblical literature as studied by Old Testament scholars. See Murray below and also the essays in Bernhard/Anderson (ed.) (1984) *Creation in the Old Testament.* London: SPCK.

7 Nicholas Lash (1988) *Easter in Ordinary: Reflections on Human Experience and the Knowledge of God.* London: SCM, p. 232.

8 Andrew Louth (1984) 'The mysterious leap of faith' in Tom Sutcliffe and Peter Moore (eds.) *In Vitro Veritas: More Tracts for Our Times.* London: St Mary's, Bourne St, p. 89.

9 *Ibid.*, p. 91.

10 Robert Murray (1988) 'The Bible on God's world and our place in it'. *The Month*, Sept., p. 799.

11 Joni Mitchell (1969) 'Woodstock'.

4   Embryo experimentation: public policy in a pluralist society

Richard M. Hare

What is the proper relation between the moral principles that should govern public policy, including legislation, and moral principles which may be held – often passionately – by individuals, including individual legislators? The adherents of such 'personal' principles often object that proposed laws would allow people, or even compel them, to transgress the principles. Obvious examples are homosexuality and abortion law reform. People who think homosexuality an abominable sin object to the repeal of laws that make it a crime; and those who think that abortion is as wrong as murder of grown people object that a law permitting abortion in certain cases might make it permissible for other people to – as they would say – murder unborn children, or even, if they are nurses and want to keep their jobs, compel them to do so themselves.

So the question we have to consider is really this: What weight ought to be given to the objections of these people when framing and debating legislation and policy? We live in a pluralist society, which means that the moral principles held sacred among different sections of society are divergent and often conflicting; and we live in a democratic society, in which, therefore, policy and legislation have to be decided on by procedures involving voting by all of us or by our representatives; so the question becomes: What attention should we pay, whether we are legislators in parliament or simply voters in a constituency, to the personal moral opinions of other people, or even to our own? In short, how ought people's moral convictions to affect the actions done by them or by others which influence public policy?

But we cannot address this question until we have answered a prior one, namely: What consideration ought in general to be given to moral principles of any kind when framing legislation and policy? There are three positions on this which I wish to distinguish. The first two seem to me unacceptable, for reasons which I shall give. I will call the first the *Realist* or 'Keep morality out of politics' position. It holds that the function of policy and of legislation is to preserve the interests, which may be purely selfish interests, of the governed; if moral considerations seem to conflict with this function, they should be ignored. Politicians have a moral duty to subordinate, in their political actions, all *other* moral duties to that of preserving the interests of the governed. This position leaves them with just one moral duty: it treats the situation of a government in power as analogous to that of an agent (say a lawyer who might be thought by some to have a duty to preserve the interests of his client even at the cost of ignoring some other supposed moral duties).

The difficulty with this position is that no reason is given by its advocates why that should be the politician's supreme and only duty. When a moral question is in dispute, as this one certainly is, we need some method, other than appeals to the convictions of those who maintain the position, of deciding whether to believe them or not. I shall therefore postpone discussion of this position until we are in possession of such a method, which will be after we have examined the third position.

The second position goes to the opposite extreme from the first. It holds that morality does apply to political actions and to legislation (very much so). The way it applies is this: there are perfect laws (laid up in Heaven as it were), to which all human laws ought morally to be made to conform. There are various versions of this position, which I shall call generically the *Natural Law* position, although that expression also has other different uses. One version says that there is a moral law and that the function of ordinary positive laws is to copy this and add appropriate penalties and sanctions. Thus murder is wrong according to the moral law, and the function of positive law and the duty of the legislators are to make it illegal and impose a penalty.

According to this version all sins ought to be made crimes. But there is a less extreme version according to which not all ought to be: there are some actions which are morally wrong but which the law ought not to intervene to punish. For example in many societies adultery is held to be wrong but is not a criminal offence. And it may be further added that not all crimes have to be sins. If the law requires people always to carry an identity card, I may be subject to penalties if I do not, but many people would not want to say that I am *morally* at fault. But it does not follow from my not being morally at fault if I break the law that the legislators were morally at fault when they made the law. They might have had very good reasons – even good moral reasons – for making the law (for example that it would facilitate the apprehension of criminals). A distinction is thus made between what are called *mala in se* (acts wrong in themselves) and *mala prohibita* (acts wrong only because they have been made illegal).

The trouble with this position is very similar to that with the first and extreme opposite position. No way has been given of telling what is in the natural law, nor of telling what sins ought to be made crimes, and which crimes are also sins. That is why, when appeal is made to the natural law, or to a moral law to which positive laws morally ought to be made to conform, people disagree so radically about what in particular this requires legislators to do. To quote the great Danish jurist Alf Ross, 'Like a harlot, the natural law is at the disposal of everyone' (1958, p. 261). Here again we shall have to postpone discussion until we have a safe method of handling such questions as 'How do we decide rationally, and not merely by appeal to prejudices dignified by the name of "deep moral convictions", what legislators morally ought to do?'

There is another, more serious, thing wrong with the second or Natural Law position. It assumes without argument that the only moral reason for passing laws is that they conform to the natural law. But there can be many reasons other than this why laws ought to be passed. If, for example, it is being debated whether the speed limit on motorways ought to be raised or lowered, the argument is not about whether it is in accordance with the moral or natural law that people should drive no faster than a certain speed. There may, certainly, be moral reasons, irrespective of any law, why people ought not to drive faster than, or slower than, a certain speed on certain roads at certain times and under certain traffic and weather conditions. But that is not what legislators talk about. They talk about what the *consequences* of having a certain law would be. For example, they ask what effect a lower limit would have on the overall consumption or conservation of fuel; what the effect would be in total on the accident figures; whether a higher limit would make it necessary to adopt a higher and therefore more costly specification for the design of motorways; whether a lower limit would lead to widespread disregard of and perhaps contempt for the law; and so on. What they are asking, as responsible legislators, is not whether 70 or 80 mph conforms to the natural law, but what they would be doing, i.e. bringing about, if they passed a certain law.

And this requirement to consider what one is doing does not apply only to the decisions of legislators. What I have said responsible legislators do is what all responsible agents have to do if they are to act morally. To act is to do something, and the morality of the act depends on what one is doing. And what one is doing is bringing about certain changes in the events that would otherwise have taken place – altering the history of the universe in a certain respect. For example, if in pulling the trigger I would be causing someone's death, that is a different act from what it would be if I pointed my gun at the ground; and the difference is morally relevant. The difference in the morality of the acts is due to a difference in what I would be causing to happen if I tightened my finger on the trigger. This does not imply that I am responsible for *all* the consequences of my bodily movements. There are well canvassed exceptions (accident, mistake, unavoidable ignorance, etc.), and there are many consequences of my bodily movements that I cannot know of and should not try to, such as the displacement of particular molecules of air. Only some, not all, of the consequences are morally relevant (see Hare, 1981, pp. 62ff. and references). But when allowance has been made for all this, what I am judged on morally is what I bring about.

It is sometimes held that we are only condemned for doing something when we *intend* to do it. This is right, properly understood. If we are judging the moral character of an agent, only what he does intentionally is relevant. But it is wrong to think that we can circumscribe intentions too narrowly for this purpose. There is a distinction, important for some purposes, between direct and oblique intentions (see Bentham, 1789, ch. 8, section 6; Hart, 1967). To intend some consequence directly one has to desire it. To intend it obliquely one has only to foresee it. But in the present context it is important that oblique intentions as well as direct intentions are relevant to the morality of actions. We have the duty to avoid bringing about consequences that we ought not to bring about, even if we do not desire those consequences in themselves, provided only that we know that they will be consequences. I am to blame if I knowingly bring about someone's death in the course of some plan of mine, even if I do not desire his death in itself – that is, even if I intend the death only obliquely and not directly. As we shall see, this is very relevant to the decisions of legislators (many of whose intentions are oblique), in that they have a duty to consider consequences of their legislation that they can foresee, and not merely those that they desire.

The legislators are to be judged morally on what they are doing (i.e. bringing about) by passing their laws. They will be condemned morally, in the speed limit example, if they make the limit so high that the accident rate goes up significantly, or so low that it is universally disregarded and unenforceable and, as a result, the law is brought into disrespect. And this brings me to my third possible position on the question of how morality applies to law-making. I will call it the *Consequentialist* position. It says that legislators, if they want to make their acts as legislators conform to morality (that is, to pass the laws they morally ought to pass and not those they ought not) they should look at what they would be doing if they passed them or threw them out. And this means, what changes in society or in its environment they would be bringing about.

What legislators are doing, or trying to do, is to bring about a certain state of society rather than some other, so far as the law can effect this – that is, a state of society in which certain sorts of things happen. The legislators are not going themselves to be doing any of these things directly, although, as I have been maintaining, they will be bringing it about intentionally that the things happen, and the bringing about is an act of theirs. There is a school of casuistry which holds that we are not to be held responsible for things which other people do as a result of what we do. I do not think that this school can have anything to say about the question we are considering. For *everything* that happens as a result of the laws that the legislators pass is something that other people do. In the narrow sense in which these casuists use the word 'do' the legislators do nothing except pass the laws. So on this view the legislators are simply not to be held responsible for anything that happens in society; so far as morality goes they can do as they please. I shall therefore say no more about this school of casuistry.

Consequentialism as a theory in moral philosophy, which I have been advocating, has received a lot of hostile criticism in recent years. This is because people have not understood what the consequentialist position is. I do not see how anybody could deny the position I have just outlined, because to deny it is to deny that what we are judged morally for (what we are responsible for) is our actions, i.e. what we bring about. What makes people look askance at what they call consequentialism is the thought that it might lead people to seek good consequences at the cost of doing what is morally wrong – as it is said, to do evil that good may come. But this is a misunderstanding. It would indeed be possible to bring about *certain* desirable consequences at the cost of bringing about certain *other* consequences which we ought not to bring about. But if the whole of the consequences of our actions (what in sum we do) were what we ought to do, then we must have acted rightly, all things considered.

There is also a further misconception. People sometimes speak as if there were a line to be drawn between an action in itself, and the consequences of the action. I am not saying that according to some ways of speaking such a line cannot be drawn; but only that it is not going to divide the morally relevant from the morally irrelevant. In the 'gun' example, nobody would wish to say that my victim's death, which is an intended consequence of my pulling the trigger, is irrelevant to the morality of my act, and that only the movement of my finger is relevant. I intend both, and, as I have said, what I intend obliquely is relevant to the morality of the act as well as what I intend directly. There are a lot of questions, interesting to philosophers of action, which could be gone into here; but I have said enough for the purposes of the present argument.

It is now time to look again at the first two positions I distinguished. What is wrong with both of them is that they ignore what the third position rightly takes into account, namely the consequences of legislation and policy, that is, what the legislators and policy-makers are *doing* by their actions. In short, both these positions encourage irresponsibility in governments. The first position, indeed, does impose on governments a moral duty of responsibility so far as the interests of their subjects go. But what about the effects of their actions on the rest of the world? Ought the British government not to have thought about the interests of Australians when it arranged its notorious atomic tests at Maralinga? Ought it not now to think about acid rain in Norway when regulating power station emissions? Hitler, perhaps, was a good disciple of this position when he thought just about the interests of Germans and said 'Damn the rest'. If we are speaking of moral duties, surely governments have duties to people in other countries. What these duties are, and how they are to be reconciled with duties to the governments' own citizens, is a subject that is fortunately outside the scope of this paper. I shall consider only what duties governments and legislators have in relation to the states of their own societies which they are by their actions bringing about.

What I have called the Natural Law position is even more open to the charge of irresponsibility. It says that there are model laws laid up in heaven, and that the legislators have a duty to write these into the positive law of the land no matter what the consequences may be for those who have to live under them. This might not be so bad if we had any way of knowing what was in the model code. But we have not; all we have is a diversity of moral convictions, differing wildly from one another, without any reasons being given by those who hold them why we should agree with them. That is one of the facts of life in a pluralist society. So what happens in practice is that people set up pressure groups (churches are ready-made pressure groups, and there are others on both sides of most disputes), and produce rhetoric and propaganda in attempts to bounce the legislators into adopting their point of view. It cannot be denied that in the course of this exercise useful arguments may be produced on both sides. But when the legislators come to their own task, which is to decide what they morally ought to do, we could wish that they had more to go on than a lot of conflicting propaganda. There ought to be a way in which they can think about such matters rationally, and decide for themselves what they really ought to do. This is especially to be hoped for when they are deciding about embryo experimentation.

Commissions and committees that are set up to help governments decide such questions are often no help at all. If, like the Glover working party (1989), they examine and assess the arguments on both sides and clarify the issues between them, they can be of great help. If, on the other hand, like the Warnock Committee (1984), they simply repeat the intuitions that are current, without going carefully into the arguments that might support them, they will not much enlighten the public discussions

(Hare, 1987). It is plain that the latter procedure will not do as a means of arriving at rational guidance for governments on moral questions affecting policy. Suppose we were to try this method in a committee in, say, South Africa. A lot of people in South Africa think it is immoral for blacks to swim even in the same private pool, let alone on the same public beach, as whites. So, if a lot of such people found themselves on a government committee about racial policy with somebody of Mary Warnock's philosophical views presiding, the committee would certainly and unanimously recommend the retention of 'whites only' beaches, and would not think it necessary to give any but the most perfunctory reasons. This is simply a recipe for the perpetuation of prejudices without having to justify them. And it is what has happened frequently on committees about IVF, surrogacy, embryo experimentation and the like.

All who handle or advise on such questions ought to be looking for arguments and testing them. So the next thing we need to ask is: What makes an argument on this sort of topic a good one? The answer has been anticipated in what I have said already. Reasoning about moral questions should start by asking what we would be doing if we followed a certain proposal. And what we would be doing is bringing about certain consequences. So what we have to ask first is: What consequences would we be bringing about if we followed it? That is what any responsible government, and any responsible committee advising a government, has to ask first.

It is not, of course, the last thing that they have to ask. They have then to go on to ask which of these consequences are ones that they morally ought to be trying to bring about and which not. But at least they will have made a good start if they have tried to find out what the consequences would be. The question of embryo experimentation illustrates this very well. This has been as vexed a question in Australia as in Britain. Suppose that Australian legislators are persuaded by one of the pressure groups in this field, or by the Tate Committee (1986), that they ought to ban all embryo experimentation, and proceed to do so. One consequence is likely to be that the advance of technology in this field will be retarded by the cessation of such experiments, at least in Australia. Perhaps the scientists will get jobs elsewhere in order to continue their experiments; but perhaps, if other governments are taking or likely to take the same line, they will find it difficult to do so. So there will be the further result that the benefits that could come from the research (for example, help to infertile couples to have children, or the elimination of some crippling hereditary diseases) will not be realized.

I have given the strongest arguments on one side. What are those on the other? We might start by thinking that a further consequence of the legislation will be that a lot of embryos will survive which otherwise would not have survived (assuming for simplicity that, as is probably the case, nearly all experiments on embryos using present techniques involve the subsequent death of the embryo). But actually that is wrong: the consequence will not be that embryos survive – at least not in all cases. Whether it is will depend on whether the embryos in question are so-called 'spare' embryos, or embryos created specially for experimentation. If they are spare embryos, indeed, the consequence of the legislation will be that they will survive *the threat of experimentation*. But if we ask what will happen to them if they survive this threat, the answer will be that either a home will be found for them and they will be implanted (perhaps after a period in the freezer) or they will perish, because there is nothing else that can be done with them. In the first case they were not really *spare* embryos. But if we assume that there are going to be at least some embryos which really are spare, and for which, therefore, no home can be found, the result of the legislation will not be different from what it would have been if there had been no legislation: they will perish just the same.

Suppose however that, faced with this argument, the legislators were to tighten up the law and say that *no* embryos were to be allowed, or caused, to perish. The consequence of this would be that no embryos would be produced artificially except those for which it was certain that a home could be found. For under such a law nobody is going to produce embryos knowing that no homes can be found for them, and that therefore he (or she) will end up in court. So the consequence of this tighter law will be that those embryos will not be produced in the first place.

The same is true of embryos produced especially for research. The result of a ban on such research will be that embryos for whom a home is in prospect will be produced and implanted, but that those (whether spare or specially created for experimentation) for whom there is no hope of implantation will simply not be produced at all. The legislators, in making the decision whether to impose such a ban on experimentation or not, are in effect deciding whether to make it the case that these embryos perish, or to make it the case that they never come into existence at all.

It is not in point here to argue whether the intentions of the experimenter (to kill or to let die, or not to produce in the first place, for example) make a difference to the morality of *his* (or *her*) actions, or to our assessment of *his* moral character. That is not what we are talking about. We are talking about the morality of the *legislators'* actions, and possibly also about *their* moral character (though it is not clear whether the latter should concern us – the fact that the moral character of some legislators is past praying for does not affect the morality of the legislation they vote for). We are talking about the morality of the actions of the legislator, not of the experimenter, and it is the consequences (the intended consequences) of the legislation that affect this. And since it is the consequences to the embryo and to the grown person that the embryo might turn into which are thought to be relevant here, and the legislation makes no significant difference to these, I shall be arguing that such considerations provide no argument for banning the experimentation: no argument to set against the arguments for allowing it that I have already mentioned.

Suppose then that we try to look at the question from the embryo's point of view (though actually, as we shall see, the embryo does not *have* a point of view, and this is important). The alternatives for the embryo are two: never to have existed, and to perish. I cannot see that, if we take the liberty of allowing the embryo a point of view, the embryo will find anything to choose between these two alternatives, because in any case embryos know nothing about what happens to them. So the legislation makes no difference to the embryo. For an ordinary grown human being, by contrast, there is a big difference between never having existed and perishing, because perishing is usually an unpleasant and often a painful process, and frustrates desires for what we might have done if we had not perished. But for the embryo it is not unpleasant to perish, and it has no desires.

I conclude that from the point of view of these embryos (namely those for whom the alternatives are as I have described) the legislation makes no difference. But now what about the point of view of the grown person that the embryo might develop into if it were implanted? That grown person certainly would have a point of view; he (or she) would have desires and would not want to perish now that he was grown up. But is there any difference, for this grown person, between not having been produced as an embryo in the first place and, after having been produced, perishing before achieving sentience? I cannot see any; so it is hard to avoid the conclusion that the legislation makes no difference to the grown person either.

The Tate Committee, rightly in my opinion, attached great importance to the *potential* that the embryo has of becoming a grown person (1986, pp. 8 and 25). But it drew what seems to me the wrong conclusion from this potential. What makes the potential of the embryo important is that if it is not realized, or is frustrated, there will not be that grown person. But if, as in the cases we are considering, there will not be that grown person anyway, how is the potential important? Indeed, *is* there really any potential? That is, if what is important is the possibility (this word is to be preferred to 'potential') of producing that grown person, and there is no such possibility (because the legislators have a choice between either doing something that will result in the embryo that would develop into that grown person not existing, or doing something that will result in it perishing) it looks as if the legislators can forget about *this* reason for imposing a ban on experimentation. For a possible explanation of why the Tate Committee was led into this false move, see Buckle (1988).

It seems therefore as if the reason we have been considering in favour of a ban, namely that it is necessary in order to save the lives of embryos, falls down; for this is only a reason if thereby the possibility of there being those grown people is preserved, and in these cases this is not so. They are analogous to a case in which the embryo has a defect because of which it is sure to perish before it develops into a baby; in *that* case is there any moral reason for preserving it? They are also analogous to the case where because of 'cleavage arrest' (see Dawson, 1988) there is no hope of the embryo ever becoming a child; such embryos just stop developing, and in the present state of *in vitro* technology nothing can be done to start development up again. It is hard to see what is lost if such embryos with no potentiality for turning into babies are destroyed, since they will perish anyway; and it is just as hard to see why the same does not apply to other embryos with no hope of survival.

But the preservation of the embryo is the main – indeed the only significant – reason given for imposing a ban; and since, so far as I can see, the reasons given on the opposite side, also concerned with the consequences of imposing it, are much more cogent, and affect many more lives much more powerfully (the lives of those who will be given children if the experiment leads to advances in techniques, the lives of those children themselves, and the lives of those who will otherwise suffer from genetic defects which research could help eliminate), I conclude that rational and responsible legislators would not impose a ban, and that clear-headed committees who could tell the difference between a good and a bad argument would not recommend it. I give this as an illustration of how those concerned with such questions should reason about them. The same method works for other questions in this field, such as surrogacy and IVF by donor, and indeed for the whole question of whether *all* artificial methods of reproduction should be banned, as the Vatican (1987) seems to think. But I have had to be content with an illustration.

To put the matter bluntly: we should stop wasting our breath on the question of when human life begins. Even if we grant for the sake of argument that it begins at fertilization (however that is defined) – even if we grant that there is a continuity of individual human existence from that time, so that I can answer Professor Anscombe's (1985) strikingly phrased question 'Were you a zygote?' in the affirmative – it is going to make no difference to the moral question of what the law ought to be on embryo experimentation. For imagine that I am a grown person who was once a zygote produced by IVF. In that case, I am certainly very glad that I was produced, and that nobody destroyed me, or for that matter the gametes that turned into me. But if you ask me whether I wish there had been a law at that time forbidding embryo experimentation, I answer that I am glad there was no such law. For if there had been, then very likely the IVF procedure which produced me would never have been invented. And such a law could not, in principle, have done anything for me. For though, if I had come into existence, it would have prevented my being destroyed, it would also have made false the antecedent of this hypothetical: I never would have come into existence in the first place.

I have spoken generally throughout of the embryo and the grown person, and not mentioned much the stages in between, such as the foetus, the neonate and the child. This is because the point I have been trying to make can be made clearly for the two extreme cases. What implications all this has for neonates and foetuses – and for that matter for pairs of gametes before fertilization – requires further discussion. But it is a big step towards clarity if we can see that at any rate in the case of the embryo it simply does not matter morally whether, or at what point in time, it became an individual human being. What matters is what we are doing to the person, in the ordinary sense of 'person', that the embryo will or may turn into.

REFERENCES

This chapter is reprinted from *Bioethics News* 7, 1987. It is also published in Kuhse H. and Singer P. (eds.) (1990) *Embryo Experimentation*, Cambridge University Press and Hare (1993) *Essays on Bioethics*, Oxford University Press.

Anscombe, G. E. M. (1985) 'Were you a zygote?' in A. P. Griffiths (ed.) *Philosophy and Practice*. Royal Institute of Philosophy Lectures 19, supplement to *Philosophy* 59. Cambridge University Press

Bentham, J. (1789) *An Introduction to the Principles of Morals and Legislation*. London: T. Payne and Sons

Buckle, S. (1988) 'Arguing from potential'. *Bioethics* 2. Reprinted in Kuhse and Singer (eds.) (1990) *Embryo Experimentation*. Cambridge University Press

Dawson, K. (1988) 'Segmentation and moral status *in vivo* and *in vitro*: a scientific perspective'. *Bioethics* 2. Reprinted in Kuhse and Singer (eds.) (1990)

Glover, J. C. B. (chair) (1989) *Fertility and the Family*, Report of EC Working Party. Fourth Estate

Hare, R. M. (1981) *Moral Thinking*. Oxford University Press

(1987) 'IVF and the Warnock Report' in Chadwick R. (ed.) *Ethics, Reproduction and Genetic Control*. London: Routledge. Reprinted in Hare (1993)

(1988), 'Possible people', *Bioethics* 2. Reprinted in Hare (1993)

(1993), *Essays on Bioethics*. Oxford University Press

Hart, H. L. A. (1967) 'Intention and punishment'. *Oxford Review* no. 4. Reprinted in Hart (1968) *Essays in the Philosophy of Law*: Oxford University Press

Ross, A. (1958) *On Law and Justice (Om ret og retfaerdighed)*. Trans. M. Dutton. London: Stevens

Tate, M. (chair) (1986) *Human Embryo Experimentation in Australia*. Senate Select Committee. Canberra: Australian Government Publication Service

Vatican (1987) 'Congregation for the doctrine of the faith', *Instruction on Respect for Human Life in its Origin and on the Divinity of Procreation: Replies to Certain Questions of the Day*. Vatican City

Warnock, Baroness M. (chair) (1984) *Report of Committee of Inquiry into Human Fertilization and Embryology*. HMSO, cmnd. 9314. Reprinted (1985) as *A Question of Life*, with new introduction and conclusion. Oxford: Blackwell

5   Ethical considerations in genetic testing: an empirical study of presymptomatic diagnosis of Huntington's disease

Jason Brandt

Advances in molecular biology have given rise to a new era in medical diagnostics. Physicians will soon be able to detect many serious diseases, or determine high genetic risk for them, years before symptom onset. Prenatal and presymptomatic genetic tests already exist for several single-gene illnesses, including Duchenne muscular dystrophy, cystic fibrosis, polycystic kidney disease, and Huntington's disease. Tests indicating susceptibility to certain forms of cancer, heart disease, Alzheimer's disease, bipolar affective disorder, alcoholism, and other common illnesses are likely to be developed in the not-too-distant future.

Although predictive DNA tests have the potential to revolutionize the practice of medicine, their social, economic, and ethical complexities are only now beginning to be seriously addressed (Holtzman, 1989). This chapter will outline some of the ethical issues involved in predictive genetic testing, and illustrate them with examples from a program of testing for Huntington's disease at the Johns Hopkins University School of Medicine. One of the primary objectives of this program is to provide sound empirical data to serve as a basis for ethical decision making in the area of genetic diagnosis.

The decision to be tested

Under virtually all circumstances, informed consent should be obligatory in genetic testing of adults for future disease vulnerability. The reasons for this are several. First, predictive genetic tests represent a new and innovative, if not experimental, technology. They are not yet part of routine clinical practice, and our experience with them is limited. Secondly, such tests are inherently elective and discretionary. At least currently, one cannot easily conceive of a test for future disease susceptibility being a necessary intervention in a medical emergency or for public safety. Finally, and perhaps most significantly, the effects of such testing on individuals are largely unknown. The psychological and social consequences to a currently healthy person of finding out that he or she carries a latent genetic defect (and, possibly, that the defect has been passed on to offspring) have not yet been determined. We might expect that some proportion of test-takers will respond poorly to receiving such news. A morbid response can, of course, be defined in a number of ways, but suicide, severe emotional distress, marital and family discord, abuse of drugs, and severe impairments in role responsibilities (e.g. difficulties at work) are the potential outcomes most often discussed. For all these reasons, those opting to be tested should be made aware of the potential hazards of testing, as well as the potential benefits. They should be assisted by knowledgeable clinicians in deciding whether the potential benefits justify the risks.

Having argued that informed consent is a *necessary* condition for genetic testing, one might ask whether it is a *sufficient* condition. In other words, is it ever ethically justified to deny testing to anyone? Our position has been that if one could reasonably expect that testing someone for a latent genetic defect would result in serious harm to that person or others, then, depending on the circumstances (e.g. if there is virtual certainty that grave harm will be done, or if the person's choice is not truly autonomous), one would be ethically justified in refusing to test that individual. Thus, for example, the refusal of testing to an unstable person who expressed an intent to commit suicide in the event of a positive test would be an ethical action.

In some ways, the clinician who decides that he or she will not perform a genetic test is making the type of judgment that is routine in medical practice. There are few, if any, diagnostic or therapeutic procedures that are available "on demand." A patient who walks into a neurologist's office requesting a head CT scan because of severe headaches is in no sense ethically "entitled" to have the procedure done. While he or she might ultimately receive such a scan, it is not before the physician performs an examination and exercises considerable professional judgment. Similarly, plastic (reconstructive) surgeons carefully evaluate patients' motives and expectations of results before performing elective cosmetic surgery.

Implications for the family

In discussions of ethical issues in presymptomatic genetic testing, parallels are often drawn with other sorts of controversial biomedical tests: those for HIV antibodies, for example, or for drug metabolites in urine. One characteristic of predictive genetic tests that sets them apart from other diagnostic procedures is that the results of such tests typically have very substantial, direct implications for others in the family and for future generations. The potential for conflict between the interests of the individual and the interests of his or her relatives is significant.

Genetic linkage tests, such as the one currently available for Huntington's disease, determine genetic risk for an individual by tracking the presence of a disease-linked characteristic (often a particular pattern in the DNA) in relatives affected with the disease and its absence in unaffected relatives. These tests require the cooperation of many family members and require that certain assumptions be made about the accuracy of pedigree information. They assume, for example, that relatives of the consultand can unambiguously be determined to be affected or unaffected by the disorder in question. This can be especially problematic for psychiatric disorders, where the same genetic defect may result in different phenotypes or may not be fully expressed. The need to have relatives examined by expert diagnosticians in order to offer a predictive test to someone at risk might lead the consultand, together with the testing facility, to adopt manipulative and even coercive measures to get uncooperative relatives diagnosed. DNA samples also are needed from multiple family members, including those who may be reluctant to be involved in such a testing procedure.

Genetic linkage tests also assume reliable paternity information. If the fatherhood information provided is incorrect, both false positive and false negative errors may occur. Occasionally, false paternity will be detected by linkage analysis, even when paternity is not tested explicitly. An unresolved ethical issue in genetic testing is whether it is appropriate for such information to be disclosed to the individual requesting testing, thereby risking significant family turmoil, when he or she has not asked for that information.

Obligations to respect the privacy of patients and the confidentiality of professional–patient communication dictate that the results of predictive genetic tests be disclosed only to the individual tested, and not to others in the family without the patient's permission. One might easily imagine a scenario, however, where the spouse or an adult child of someone undergoing genetic testing wants to know the results for his or her own benefit or the benefit of other family members. For example, it might be argued that the wife of a man genetically tested has a legitimate need for the test results, especially if the couple is planning to have children. Not disclosing this information might cause her great emotional harm, and possibly physical and psychological harm to future children. In such circumstances, does the clinician have the moral right, or even the moral obligation, to inform the relatives of the results without the patient's authorization? In most such conflicts, the clinician's duty to respect confidentiality and the autonomy of the patient probably supersedes any obligations he or she has to assist or prevent harm to members of the patient's family. This setting of priorities reflects the specific obligations and needs of the patient–clinician relationship, in which mutual trust and confidence is crucial. Hopefully, however, the clinician will discuss with the patient the perilous position in which he is putting his family, and work with him in attempting to reach a more satisfactory solution.

A related issue is whether it is ever permissible to deny testing to an individual if a positive test result would bring extreme hardship to his or her family. Here, the clinician must weigh his or her responsibility to the patient against that to the family. Again, this is a situation where frank discussions with the patient and the family may disclose hidden motives and reveal previously unseen solutions.

Implications for social institutions

Earlier, it was argued that informed consent was necessary for predictive genetic tests under virtually all circumstances. What, however, are the exceptions? Is it ever morally permissible to override individual autonomy and compel an individual to be tested? The most plausible case for mandatory testing would be if doing so would protect others from extreme harm. For example, it might be a justified (or indeed a morally responsible) act for a government agency to insist that commercial pilots with strong family histories of heart disease be genetically tested to determine their risk for myocardial infarction (if such a reliable test existed). Whether this constitutes an inappropriate invasion of privacy or is simply good public health policy is clearly a contentious issue.

The issues of confidentiality discussed earlier in the context of the family are perhaps even more significant in the context of the interests of corporations and other organizations. Rules of privacy and confidentiality would appear to dictate that employers, insurance companies, and other third-party payers for health care not have independent access to test results. However, it has been argued (Quarrell et al., 1989) that access to genetic information by insurance companies is appropriate, since the entire insurance industry rests on accurate assignment of individuals to risk categories. At the same time, those in greatest need of insurance protection may be denied coverage (or affordable coverage) if insurance carriers are allowed access to test results (Brandt et al., 1989a). A related difficult issue is whether an insurance company should be permitted to make genetic testing a precondition for issuance of an insurance policy. Such a requirement would clearly be to the financial advantage of the insurance company and would probably result in lower premiums for those who have no detectable genetic vulnerabilities. The number of such people is likely to dwindle, however, as efforts to map the human genome proceed and the number of identified disease-promoting genes increases.

There appears to be significant public support for genetic testing and genetic engineering, as long as they are limited to the diagnosis and prevention of disease and the results are not used by employers, insurance companies, or governments. In a poll of 1,254 US adults (*Business Week*, November 18, 1985), 50 percent of those questioned said they would take genetic tests which determined whether they would develop incurable and fatal diseases later in life, if such tests were available. Only 11 percent, however, believed that employers should have the right to require such tests before hiring someone, and only 21 percent believed that insurance companies would be justified in refusing to insure the lives or health of those who test positive for genes causing fatal illnesses. Sixty-four percent of those queried believed that altering genes to cure fatal diseases should be allowed, while only 9 percent would be interested in gene manipulation to have smarter, physically stronger, or more attractive children.

Currently, most genetic testing is individual and family based. Whether such testing should ever become population based, leading to large-scale genetic screening programs, is an important question to consider. At the present time, most DNA linkage tests are too cumbersome methodologically and too expensive for wide-scale use. However, methods are being streamlined and costs will probably be declining as the technology evolves. Although genetic screening programs certainly hold promise for detecting genetic anomalies, they may do so at the expense of individual privacy.

Implementation of a predictive testing program for Huntington's disease

Some of the issues discussed thus far are being confronted currently in the program of predictive testing for Huntington's disease at the Johns Hopkins University School of Medicine. Huntington's disease is a degenerative neuropsychiatric disorder characterized by involuntary choreiform movements (jerking and writhing), impaired voluntary movements, progressive loss of cognitive abilities, and emotional symptoms, including depression, apathy, and irritability. The disease is caused by a single dominant gene. Any man or woman who has an affected parent has a 50 percent chance of developing the condition. Onset of the disease is insidious, usually beginning between ages 35 and 45, past the typical age of childbearing. Although palliative treatments exist, the progression is inexorable and the disease is incurable. There are approximately 25,000 patients with the disorder in the United States, and approximately 125,000 individuals are at 50 percent risk (Folstein, 1989).

In 1983, a genetic marker for Huntington's disease was discovered by Gusella and associates (Gusella *et al.*, 1983). This marker is a region on chromosome 4 that is very close to the Huntington's disease gene. Although not the gene itself, this DNA marker is so close to the gene that its presence indicates a 95 percent or greater chance of the latter also being inherited. The discovery of this marker permitted the development of a genetic linkage test with high predictive value for those at-risk individuals with affected relatives. If a healthy at-risk person inherits the marker from his affected parent, he has a 95 percent or greater chance of having inherited the Huntington's disease gene and hence developing the illness. Upon discovery of the marker for Huntington's disease, clinicians and researchers began planning for ways to offer a predictive test in a socially and morally responsible way.

Some have argued that such a test should not be performed at all. First, there is currently no cure for Huntington's disease. Some of the choreiform movements and emotional symptoms can be treated pharmacologically, but the overall course of the disorder is not affected. Where is the wisdom in early diagnosis, one might ask, when it cannot lead to early intervention? Secondly, there is the potential for significant psychological and social morbidity after such a test. There is already a high prevalence of psychological disorders (especially affective disorder) in persons at risk for Huntington's disease (Folstein *et al.*, 1983b), and the suicide rate in patients is approximately four times the population rate (Farrer, 1986). Thirdly, the disease often has a late onset. Is it reasonable to compromise an individual's enjoyment of what could otherwise be many years of healthy, productive life with the foreknowledge that she will develop symptoms when she reaches age 40 and will live another 10 to 20 years? Finally, the test is less than 100 percent accurate. As already noted, the original marker permitted a test that was only 95 percent accurate. More tightly linked markers have since been isolated, allowing tests with up to 99 percent diagnostic accuracy (Gilliam *et al.*, 1987; Hayden *et al.*, 1988; Wasmuth *et al.*, 1988). Still, one might argue that it would be better to wait until the gene itself is isolated, enabling a less cumbersome test with perfect predictive value (barring laboratory error).

At the same time, the majority of people at risk for the illness are favorably inclined toward presymptomatic testing. Surveys of young at-risk adults have indicated that 60 to 80 percent think predictive testing is a good idea and would take a safe and reliable test (Mastromauro *et al.*, 1987; Stern and Eldridge, 1975; Tyler and Harper, 1983). Some individuals report that a test would allow them to make more informed decisions concerning childbearing, careers, education, and family finances. Many at-risk people say that a test result, *any* test result, would give them some relief from the anxiety associated with not knowing. Furthermore, some say that the imperfect linkage test now available is preferable to waiting for a direct gene test. A more perfect test – one that is informative for everyone and without a margin of error – would leave no hope for those who test positive.

The staff of the Huntington's Disease Center at the Johns Hopkins University School of Medicine adopted the position that the currently available test has sufficient potential to improve the lives of some people at risk that it should be made available to those who feel they would benefit. Since there was no empirical basis from which to predict the psychosocial effects of testing, the decision was made to conduct the test in a closely monitored way, with the psychosocial effects carefully studied. The technology might be well established, but the best mechanism for implementing that technology as a clinical test is unknown. Predictive testing was thus initiated in September 1986 as a program of empirical psychological research. The program was funded by the National Institutes of Health, and later by the Huntington's Disease Society of America and the National Institute of Mental Health. The research protocol, especially the methods for protecting the well-being of tested subjects, underwent close scrutiny by the Johns Hopkins Joint Committee on Clinical Investigation and by the funding agencies. Two senior clinicians (professors of psychiatry and medicine) with major interests in the ethics of clinical research agreed to serve as ethics consultants to the project. They were consulted as needed to help decide what course of action was appropriate in especially difficult cases.

The first goal of the testing program was to educate potential test-takers about the test and the research program. Letters inviting at-risk persons and their relatives to attend educational sessions were sent to 387 people at risk for Huntington's disease who were known to our Center and who lived within commuting distance (Quaid *et al.*, 1989). While only 47 at-risk persons attended one of the group sessions (accompanied by 54 non-at-risk family members), many more have since requested testing. During the educational sessions, the technical aspects of the test were described in non-technical language, making extensive use of diagrams and analogies. The limitations of the test, its error rate, and the potential psychological effects of testing were all discussed. The voluntary nature of the test was reiterated several times.

The educational sessions were found to be effective in teaching at-risk people about the test (Quaid *et al.*, 1989). Those who attended obtained higher scores on a knowledge questionnaire at the end of the session than they did before the session. More importantly, this knowledge was retained when reassessed an average of three months later, and, most importantly, was not accompanied by an increase in anxiety about testing. Although the at-risk people participating in this phase of the program represent a small and self-selected sample, our educational efforts were effective and worth the effort.

After the educational sessions were held, entry into the program began. Specific eligibility criteria were established. Each participant had to be the child of an affected patient (and therefore at 50 percent risk). Persons at 25 percent risk (those with an affected grandparent, but an as-yet unaffected parent) were not tested. One pragmatic justification for this decision is that the test is still a very limited resource and should be made available to those at greatest risk. A more important ethical consideration is that testing such a person at 25 percent risk may disclose the genetic status of his parent who is at 50 percent risk but who has not requested the presymptomatic test. Our working rule is not to test anyone if doing so imposes unsolicited information on a relative. (Recently, the protocol was modified to allow the testing of persons at 25 percent risk in such a way as *not* to reveal the status of their still-at-risk parents. Such "nondisclosing" or "exclusion" testing ascertains only whether the 25 percent risk person is actually at 50 percent risk, like his or her parent, or is at minimal [1 percent to 5 percent] risk.)

Testing is offered only to individuals over age 18. Children are not being tested because, as in most contexts, they are not regarded as competent to give independent informed consent. This research project deviated somewhat from the standard clinical practice of having parents give consent for their minor children. Our moral justification for this decision is that the procedure is of unknown "safety" and the potential risks may be substantial. In the context of biomedical research, children are often deemed especially worthy of protection from any possible harm, and it is conventional to introduce new interventions with children only after extensive testing on adults. The question remains whether it will be legitimate to test a child at a parent's request when the research stage is passed. Does a parent's right to know the future health status of a child supersede the child's right to privacy? Huntington's disease might represent a unique case, since the parent's knowledge cannot at present lead to earlier or better medical intervention.

Similarly, mentally retarded or seriously mentally ill individuals are not being tested. They, too, are considered incompetent to give truly informed consent. We have taken the position that our first responsibility is to "do no harm" and that responsibility, rather than absolute individual autonomy, prevails in deciding whether a given individual should be tested.

With this as a rule, we have postponed testing several depressed or otherwise seriously troubled individuals until their psychological disorders were appropriately treated.

Initially, individuals who lived within 150 miles of Baltimore were considered eligible for testing. The rationale for this restriction was that the ability of the project's clinical staff to intervene with psychological assistance or crisis management necessitated quick and easy access to the Center. Based on the lack of need for emergency treatment in the first three years of the program, the catchment area has recently been expanded to include all of Maryland and several nearby states.

Elaborate and specific informed consent procedures were established. Participants received extensive teaching about the test before they committed themselves to proceed. Seven separate consent procedures covered the donation of blood samples for DNA extraction, the use of the DNA to establish the linkage of new markers, the use of the DNA to test a relative, disclosure of predictive test results, and prenatal testing.

Test procedures

A baseline assessment was made of everyone who requested presymptomatic testing. For at-risk persons not previously known to our program, a detailed interview was conducted during the first visit to establish the family history of Huntington's disease and to draw the pedigree. Medical and other records were sought, and documentation of age of onset of the disease in affected relatives was obtained. For all subjects, the Quantified Neurological Examination (Folstein *et al.*, 1983a) was performed to detect subtle, preclinical neurological signs. Also during this visit, a psychiatric interview using the Schedule of Affective Disorders and Schizophrenia-Lifetime Version (SADS-L) (Endicott and Spitzer, 1978) was performed to establish whether the at-risk person presently had a diagnosable psychiatric disorder that would compromise his or her ability to consent to the procedures or participate fully in the protocol. This is done both to establish eligibility for testing as well as to establish a baseline from which to ascertain the emergence of psychological symptoms. The Mini-Mental State Exam (Folstein *et al.*, 1975), a brief cognitive screening test, was given to rule out dementia or delirium. If a potential subject was found to be suffering already from Huntington's disease or a major mental illness, he or she was counseled and referred to the Huntington's Disease Clinic or another appropriate facility for treatment.

Subjects who qualified to proceed with the study were evaluated psychologically over several sessions. This evaluation included a large number of psychological tests, mood and symptom-rating scales, and personality and social functioning inventories. The hypothesis guiding the selection of these tests and procedures as baseline measures was that the impact of receiving information about one's genetic status would vary depending on family history, preexisting personality features and coping style, psychological symptoms, cognitive efficiency, life stresses, and environmental support.

Each subject participated in at least three (typically five) 90-minute individual counseling sessions with a psychologist. All sessions took place at least two weeks apart, with the total number of visits determined by individual need. The purpose of these counseling sessions was to discuss with participants the nature of the genetic linkage test, the various outcomes that might be expected, and the impact that the results of the test might have on their lives. It was explained that a chromosomal marker for the Huntington's disease gene, and not the gene itself, is detected by this test. This implies that there would still be some uncertainty as to whether the defective gene had been inherited. Other potential sources of error, including inaccurate paternity information and diagnostic error (i.e. if a relative designated as affected with Huntington's disease actually had another condition) were discussed. Assistance was given in clarifying the family history, obtaining medical information from affected and unaffected relatives, and collecting the blood or tissue samples necessary for the genetic test to be performed. During each counseling session, the voluntary nature of the decision to be tested was emphasized. Informed consent was obtained prior to the testing.

Each subject undergoing testing was asked to identify an individual he or she knew well to be his or her confidant. The confidant attended a minimum of one counseling session and was required to be present at the time of disclosure of the test results. The role of the confidant is to provide emotional support to the person being tested and to serve as a liaison with the project staff. The requirement of a confidant may be considered somewhat over-protective on our part and a violation of strict confidentiality. However, we deemed it a reasonable and morally justified precaution during the research phase of testing, as it was intended solely to minimize risk of harm to tested individuals.

The availability of the project's professional staff for psychological support and assistance after testing was repeatedly emphasized. Every three months for the first year after disclosure of test results, and every six months for the next two years, follow-up visits with the project staff monitor the effects of disclosure with the standardized psychological tests and psychiatric scales. All participants were provided with a primary therapist (either a psychiatrist or a social worker) in our

Center to offer psychological support and treatment as needed after disclosure.

Among the rules that were adopted was strict confidentiality. No one other than the tested individual, his or her confidant, and some members of the research team have access to the genetic test results and other project data. Not even close relatives, including those whose test samples enabled the patient to be tested, have independent access to the results. Genetic test results are kept in locked research files, not in hospital records.

Another working rule is that if false paternity is detected in the course of genetic analysis, it is not disclosed. Patients are informed of this policy during pre-test counseling. If an affected father with Huntington's disease is found not to be the consultand's biological father, the consultand is told that the test is negative and he or she is no longer at risk. This decision was motivated by our obligation to prevent harm to the patient, and to keep confidential this sensitive information.

The study sample

In the first four years of the program, 152 people at risk who wanted to know their genetic status entered the study. Of these, 20 were found to be already mildly affected at entry, were diagnosed, and referred to our Huntington's Disease Clinic. As of August 1990, tests have been completed for 85 people, with the remainder still undergoing baseline testing and counseling. Of the 69 informative tests, 18 were positive for one or more linked markers (i.e. the individuals tested will almost certainly develop Huntington's disease) and 51 were negative.

The two groups of subjects with informative tests were subjected to close scrutiny to determine whether any baseline characteristics distinguished those who would test positive from those who would test negative. The marker-negative subjects were older; this is to be expected, since the longer an at-risk person remains asymptomatic, the less likely it is that he or she possesses the Huntington's disease gene. The groups did not differ in any other sociodemographic characteristic, number of minor neurological abnormalities, or score on any of the psychological tests.

Outcomes of genetic testing

At disclosure of test results, reactions ranged from joy and relief to sadness and demoralization. Presumably due to the extensive pre-test counseling, only one participant was "shocked" by the outcome, and only

Table 1. *Life events after disclosure of presymptomatic test results.*

	Marker-positive	Marker-negative
N	18	38
Mean duration of follow-up	18.17 months	21.16 months
No. of marriages	1	2
No. of children born	0	5
No. of job promotions and advancements	15	19
	(11 people)	(12 people)
No. of marital separations and divorces	2	2
No. of job losses and demotions	10	7
	(3 people)	(5 people)
No. of psychiatric hospitalizations	1	0
No. of suicide attempts	0	0

Note: Data are for marker-positive subjects (who were told their risk of developing Huntington's disease was at least 95%) and marker-negative subjects (who were told their risk was less than 5%).
*Thirteen marker-negative subjects have not yet had their first follow-up visit.

one has expressed any regret at having requested testing. In the first four years of the project, one participant who tested positive has required brief psychiatric hospitalization for depression. All the other marker-positive subjects are doing well. Table 1 summarizes some of the major life events that have occurred in the two groups of subjects. Several marker-negative subjects who remained childless before testing have since had children. The other area of greatest change has been in occupational functioning. Job successes have been proportionally more common in the marker-negative group, while job failures were more common in the marker-positive group. Psychiatric interviews and psychological testing revealed minor increases in psychological distress among those who test positive, while those who test negative experience reductions in psychological symptoms (see figure 1).

Examples of ethical problems encountered

In spite of careful planning and consideration of ethical issues, we have encountered many situations that posed ethical challenges. Some have been resolved, while others remain unresolved and subject to ongoing study. They are presented briefly below to illustrate the types of clinical decisions that must be made in actually implementing a program of presymptomatic genetic testing.

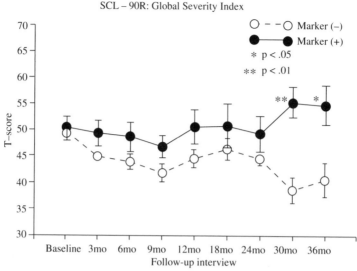

Figure 1

Global Severity Index on the Symptom Checklist (SCL – 90R) for subjects testing positive and negative for the HD marker(s) at baseline (before disclosure of test results) and at regularly-scheduled follow-up visits. (Data as of August 1990.) Subjects testing positive display a slight increase in total psychological distress, while those testing negative display a slight decrease. (50 is the average T-score; SD = 10.) Due to the variable lengths of follow-up, the number of subjects represented by each data point varies. The significant difference between the two groups at the 30-month and 36-month visits may be unreliable due to the small number of subjects represented (a total of only 8 subjects at 36 months).

Case 1:

A pair of monozygotic twins in their mid-40s is at risk for Huntington's disease. Twin A wanted to know whether she will develop Huntington's disease, while twin B did not want to know. Since offering genetic information to twin A would automatically disclose the result to twin B, the conflict here was between our desire to inform the consultand and our obligation not to inform a relative who did not want to be informed. It was explained to twin A that our working rule was to postpone testing if it would force unwanted genetic information on someone else. She was disappointed, but appreciated the predicament and understood our position. Several months later, twin B came to see us to discuss testing. She was found to be already symptomatic with the illness, meaning that twin A would also soon become affected.

Case 2:

An at-risk woman was the only member of her sibship of five to request testing. Her unaffected father believed that testing was not in the best interest of his daughter or her young family, and therefore refused to donate a blood sample. He later agreed to give a sample only if he could limit the use to which it would be put. Specifically, he was willing to cooperate in the testing of this daughter because, he said, if any of his children could handle the news, she could. However, he did not want his DNA results used to test his other children without his explicit permission. In essence, he insisted on maintaining control over his genetic material. This raises interesting ethical questions, as well as legal questions concerning proprietary rights. Who "owns" your DNA once it's in a test-tube? Who "owns" the information derived from it? After much discussion, it was decided that we would allow the father to control his level of participation in the genetic testing of his children. He donated a blood sample after he and the investigators signed an agreement specifying that results from his test would not be used in testing any of his other children without his prior written consent. Approximately one year later, another of his children requested testing and he readily agreed to use the information from his sample for this purpose.

In this same family, the first daughter expressed a strong intent to leave her husband and two small children if she tested positive for the Huntington's disease marker. She did not want them to be burdened by her, and have to endure her emotional symptoms as she had endured her mother's. In a very reasonable way, she had arranged for child care, made appropriate legal arrangements, etc. The central questions here are what qualifies as a "bad" outcome, and what (if any) is our ethical responsibility to her family? In this case, it was decided that whatever harm might be done to this woman's family if she left them was not of sufficient magnitude to exclude her from testing.

Case 3:

One young man in our project had always wanted to get his pilot's license. After testing positive for the marker linked to Huntington's disease, he became demoralized, preoccupied with his test result, and relatively uncommunicative with his wife. Six months later, he decided that if he wanted to fly, he had better do it now, and began taking flying lessons. Should he be discouraged from becoming a pilot? Would doing so be inappropriately paternalistic, or clinically responsible? If he continued to fly against our advice once symptoms began, would it be our moral or legal right, or even our duty, to report this to relevant aviation authorities? In this case, the potential for impairments in judgment, spatial perception, and motor control early in the illness was discussed with the patient, and he voluntarily discontinued the flying lessons.

Case 4:

A woman with four children of marriageable age needed blood samples from her brother and sister in order for the genetic status of her deceased, affected mother to be determined. These siblings are not in our project, and will learn nothing about their own risk. One sister, an older, married woman with no children of her own, refused to donate a blood sample. Does this sister have a moral obligation to cooperate with such testing in order to prevent harm to the next generation? Our position in such cases has been that we are very willing to discuss the testing program with reluctant relatives if they contact us, but that it would not be appropriate for us to seek out such individuals. In this case, the sister's desire not to be involved in predictive testing needed to be respected.

Case 5:

An oncology nurse at an out-of-state hospital telephoned us concerning a leukemia patient who was in need of a bone-marrow transplant and was also at risk for Huntington's disease. The physicians treating this woman were referring her to us because they wanted her tested for Huntington's disease before they performed the transplant. There appeared to be the implicit statement that they might decide not to perform this costly and risky, but life-prolonging, procedure if the test indicated that the woman would probably develop Huntington's disease. The nurse was understandably reluctant to explain or defend the request. Because the patient did not meet the eligibility criteria for our research protocol (she resided out of state and was too ill to participate in the counseling and follow-up sessions), testing was not made available to her. The major ethical question here is the weight that should be assigned someone's future disease potential when allocating scarce resources.

Case 6:

A depressed 15-year-old boy, whose father is in a nursing home with advanced Huntington's disease, was admitted to the psychiatric service of the Johns Hopkins Hospital because of school refusal, extreme irritability at home, and fears that he might become violent toward his mother. He is at risk for early onset of Huntington's disease, as his father developed the illness in his late 20s and had affective disorder early in his illness. The young man's neurological examinations were unremarkable. Since the patient's family had participated in genetic testing, samples from the patient's affected father and several other relatives had been stored and were available for use in testing. The patient's mother asked if we would test her son for the Huntington's disease marker, either with or without his knowledge. She reasoned that if he had the marker she would be more accepting of his distressing behavior and not so insistent that he attend school. If, on the other hand, he did not have the marker, she would take a stronger stance against his misbehavior. The decision was made not to test this young man, even though his mother's request was motivated by her sincere concern for his future and the implications that performing the test might have for his psychiatric treatment. Since the patient did not request testing and had not attained legal majority, he was ineligible for the research study. By virtue of his illness, he was probably also compromised in his ability to evaluate the merits of testing.

Case 7:

A woman at risk for Huntington's disease who lived in another state telephoned our Center to inform us that she was moving to Baltimore the following week to have the presymptomatic test. She had made no arrangements for housing or employment, and upon further inquiry, it became apparent that she had a very unstable past. It was suggested that she contact us after she settled in, but she demanded to be seen very shortly after arriving in town. She was living in a motel, paid for by a church-affiliated social service agency, and was being supported by newly found friends in a support group for alcoholics. During the initial interviews and examinations, she described a severely disturbed family background and personal history, which included two rapes, self-injurious behavior, anorexia and bulimia nervosa, possible alcohol abuse, and inpatient psychiatric treatment for "anger and agitation" (diagnosed as post-traumatic stress disorder and personality disorder with borderline features). Although the subject was not psychotic or otherwise incompetent to give consent for participation in the testing program, it was felt that she was so unstable, and that her social supports were so meager, that to test her would run a very high risk of precipitating a severe decompensation. The project staff felt that she should not be included in the testing program at the present time, and a similar decision was arrived at independently by our ethics consultants. The patient was told the reasons for the decision, and was informed that her case would be reconsidered in one year with no guarantees of any kind.

Case 8:

An officer in the US Army who is at risk for Huntington's disease was recently stationed in Maryland. He requested testing, but was very concerned that military authorities not find out about his risk. Since he was new to the vicinity, he did not have any close friends that he felt he could ask to be his confidant. His unaffected mother – elderly, frail, and living far away – would be the person he would choose if he were compelled to select someone. He asked that we bend the rule for him and allow him to proceed with testing without a confidant. Although we judged him to be stable and dependable enough to be tested alone if he could not find a suitable partner, we did not tell him this and instead encouraged him to continue to seek someone to accompany him through the testing process. Although he was frustrated, he stated that he understood our reason for the rule and declared his intent to hire an attorney to be his confidant. Client–attorney confidentiality, he felt, made this a safe alternative for him. Finally, however, he contacted the local chapter of the Huntington's Disease Society of America, and told his story to one of the very active and dedicated volunteers. This woman, whose own husband is in a nursing home suffering from the terminal stages of HD, became the patient's confidant. This resolution had the advantage of providing the support of someone with intimate knowledge of the disease and of facilitating contact with a community of persons facing similar decisions.

Each of these situations was handled in the context of counseling and frank discussion with the at-risk person and confidant. We attempt to avoid taking adversarial positions; we convey our concern for the person and our desire to do the right thing for all those involved, including family members. We work together with the consultand to arrive at decisions that are respectful of his or her choice, yet do not violate the rights of others and reflect our clinical judgment borne of professional training and experience.

Conclusions

The results of our pilot project thus far indicate that presymptomatic testing for Huntington's disease can be done in a manner that protects the well-being of the test takers. When provided in a context that includes extensive teaching, counseling, and follow-up, the news that one will likely develop this progressive brain disease is tolerated well, at least by our highly selected sample. We have encountered many situations that raise ethical dilemmas, but by adopting a few more-or-less common-sense principles and blending them with clinical judgment, we have been able to resolve them satisfactorily.

The fact that our testing program is a research project has afforded us some protections that a clinical testing program may not have. For example, we have not had to deal with insurance companies being asked to pay for testing, and we have been able to keep test outcomes out of official medical records. We also have had the benefit of a large, multidisciplinary team of professionals and support personnel who devote a great deal of time and energy to the testing program. Whether similar psychological outcomes will be obtained once predictive genetic tests become technically simpler and performed in environments less conducive to this level of professional involvement remains to be seen.

ACKNOWLEDGMENTS

The author is grateful for discussions with several individuals about ethical issues in DNA testing. Special thanks go to Drs. Ann-Marie Codori, David Edwin, Ruth Faden, Susan E. Folstein, Marshal F. Folstein, Thomas R. Hendrix, Haig H. Kazazian, Jr., Paul R. McHugh, Kimberly A. Quaid, and Phillip R. Slavney, although they may not agree with all the views expressed. Supported by grants NS16375, NS24841 and MH46034 from the National Institutes of Health and a grant from the Huntington's Disease Society of America.

REFERENCES

Brandt, J., Quaid, K. A. and Folstein, S. E. (1989a) 'Response to letter by Quarrell et al.'. *Journal of the American Medical Association, 262*: 2385

(1989b) 'Presymptomatic diagnosis of delayed-onset disease with linked DNA markers: The experience in Huntington's disease.' *Journal of the American Medical Association, 261*: 3108–14

Endicott, J. and Spitzer, R. L. (1978) 'A diagnostic interview: the schedule for affective disorders and schizophrenia.' *Archives of General Psychiatry, 35*: 837–44

Farrer, L. A. (1986) 'Suicide and attempted suicide in Huntington disease: implications for preclinical testing of persons at risk. *American Journal of Medical Genetics, 24*: 305–11

Folstein, M. F., Folstein, S. E. and McHugh, P. R. (1975) '"Mini-mental state": A practical method for grading the cognitive state of patients for the clinician.' *Journal of Psychiatric Research, 12*: 189–98

Folstein, S. E. (1989) *Huntington's Disease: A Disorder of Families*. Baltimore MD: Johns Hopkins University Press

Folstein, S. E., Abbott, M. H., Chase, G. A. (1983a) 'The association of affective disorder with Huntington's disease in a case series and in families.' *Psychological Medicine, 13*: 537–42

Folstein, S. E., Jensen, B., Leigh, R. J. and Folstein, M. F. (1983b) 'The measurement of abnormal movement: methods developed for Huntington's disease.' *Journal of Neurobehavioral Toxicology and Teratology, 5*: 605–9

Gilliam, T. C., Bucan, M., MacDonald, M. E. (1987) 'A DNA segment encoding two genes very tightly linked to Huntington's disease.' *Science, 238*: 950–2

Gusella, J. F., Wexler, N. S., Conneally, P. M. (1983) 'A polymorphic DNA marker linked to Huntington's disease.' *Nature, 306*: 234–8

Hayden, M. R., Robbins, C., Allard, D. (1988) 'Improved predictive testing for Huntington's disease by using three linked DNA markers.' *American Journal of Human Genetics, 43*: 689–94

Holtzman, N. A. (1989) *Proceed with Caution: Predicting Genetic Risks in the Recombinant DNA Era.* Baltimore, MD: Johns Hopkins University Press

Mastromauro, C., Myers, R. H. and Berkman, B. (1987) 'Attitudes toward presymptomatic testing in Huntington disease. *American Journal of Medical Genetics, 26:* 271–82

Quaid, K. A., Brandt, J., Faden, R. and Folstein, S. E. (1989) Knowledge, attitude, and the decision to be tested for Huntington's disease.' *Clinical Genetics, 36*: 431–8

Quaid, K. A., Brandt, J. and Folstein, S. E. (1989) 'The decision to be tested for Huntington's disease (letter).' *Journal of the American Medical Association, 257*: 3362

Quarrell, O. W. J., Bloch, M. and Hayden, M. R. (1989) 'Insurance and the presymptomatic diagnosis of delayed-onset disease (letter).' *Journal of the American Medical Association, 262*: 2384–5

Stern, R. and Eldridge, R. (1975) 'Attitudes of patients and their relatives to Huntington's disease. *Journal of Medical Genetics, 12*: 217–23

Tyler, A. and Harper, P. S. (1983) 'Attitudes of subjects at-risk and their relatives toward genetic counseling in Huntington's chorea.' *Journal of Medical Genetics, 20*: 179–88

Wasmuth, J. J., Hewitt, J., Smith, B. (1988) 'A highly polymorphic locus very tightly linked to the Huntington's disease gene.' *Nature, 332*: 734–6

6   Identity matters

Michael Lockwood

A traditional philosophical problem on which a vast amount of ink has been spilt is that of *personal identity*. John Locke, in the seventeenth century, rubbished the idea that the persistence of a person over a period of time was to be conceived as consisting in the persistence of an immaterial soul, suggesting instead that it was constituted by the later person's ability to remember actions or experiences of the earlier person:

to find wherein personal identity consists, we must first consider what *person* stands for; which I think, is a thinking intelligent being, that has reason and reflection, and can consider itself as itself, the same thinking thing, in different times and places; which it does only by that consciousness which is inseparable from thinking, and, as it seems to me, essential to it ...; and as far as this consciousness can be extended backwards to any past action or thought, so far reaches the identity of the person.[1]

As stated, Locke's precise theory generates unacceptably counterintuitive consequences, in particular that identity is nontransitive; for clearly it is possible for A to remember B's actions or experiences, and B to remember C's, without A remembering C's (if A, B and C are persons considered at different, successively earlier times). This was pointed out by Thomas Reid,[2] with his celebrated example of the elderly retired general who can remember his gallant charge as a young officer, but cannot remember, what the young officer can, being beaten, as a boy, for stealing apples: it is a manifest absurdity to say – as Locke's theory ostensibly commits him to saying – that the reminiscing retired general is the same person as the young officer leading the cavalry charge, and the young officer the same person as the boy stealing the apples, but that the general is *not* the same person as that boy. Nevertheless, it is widely believed, amongst philosophers, that Locke's approach to the problem is right in spirit. Indeed, what is perhaps the most widely discussed current approach to this issue, that of Derek Parfit in his book *Reasons and Persons*,[3] lies squarely within the Lockean tradition. Parfit describes himself as a *reductionist* about personal identity. Like Locke, he thinks that a person's identity through time is constituted by psychological links that connect later to earlier person stages, though not just memory; Parfit would also include the relation between earlier intentions and subsequent actions, the persistence of beliefs and perhaps also continuities of personality. Other philosophers have pointed out that a way of getting round the specific problem raised for Locke by Reid is to allow two person stages to constitute stages of the same person, whenever there is a chain of intermediate person stages, any two successive members of which are such that the later can remember the earlier one's actions or experiences. Parfit calls this kind of relation psychological *continuity*, generalising it to include the other sorts of link just alluded to; when any of these relations hold directly between two person stages, he says of them that they are psychologically *connected*. I shall follow this terminology in the present paper.

Anyway, there is, Parfit thinks, nothing more to our persistence through time than psychological continuity. Specifically, he holds that two person stages, A and B, are stages of the same person just in case A and B are linked by a chain of person stages any two successive members of which are *strongly* psychologically connected; that is to say, (1) enough psychological connections hold between them, (2) this connectedness is grounded in some generally reliable cause, and (3) there is no third person stage C that is linked in this fashion to A without being so linked to B, or vice versa. (This is to ensure transitivity, and has the effect of not allowing a person's identity to survive fission of the self.)

Given a pair of person stages, stages of what we would ordinarily think of as the same person, it is clear that there is a whole spectrum of degrees of psychological connectedness or continuity in which they may stand. (Typically, this connectedness is roughly a function of temporal separation, but various forms of physical or emotional trauma – a head injury, stroke or nervous breakdown – may engender a striking weakening of connectedness as between stages of the same person that are not widely separated in time.) Parfit does not want to draw from this consideration the conclusion that identity is itself a matter of degree, at least in ordinary cases, though that is a common misunderstanding of his position. Common sense would say that today's forgetful old Emeritus Professor is, after all, the same person as the young turk; and Parfit goes along with that: it will presumably be possible to decompose the Professor's life into stages successive members of which are (sufficiently) strongly connected, even if in retirement this man is far more weakly connected with the newly appointed Fellow than is the latter with the undergraduate taking Schools. Besides, ordinary usage doesn't really allow for degrees of identity: in its logic, identity is all-or-nothing. *In its logic, but not in its underlying nature.* This is the crucial point. Identity may, simply as a matter of linguistic fiat, be all-or-nothing. But what constitutes our identity is far from being all-or-nothing. And more important still, it is not, in any case, identity itself that is of moral and prudential significance here. What really matter are psychological continuity and connectedness; whatever moral and prudential significance attaches to identity derives from them.

Now this issue is of far more than merely academic interest. Questions of considerable practical importance hinge on it. Parfit himself, of course, thinks that it matters and draws from his reductionism some very sweeping moral consequences. One that Parfit mentions concerns penal justice. It is a consequence that I found myself thinking about every time Klaus Barbie appeared on my television screen during his recent trial. Clearly, a minimal necessary condition for its being just to punish a person for a crime is that the person, that very same person, committed it. Well actually I haven't the least doubt that the man sitting in the dock in Lyons (though later only briefly at the start of each day's proceedings) did do most of the beastly things of which he was accused. But Parfit forces us to ask: just how much moral force attaches to the fact (if it is a fact) that *he* did these things, given the forty-year-plus lapse of time, and its consequent erosion of psychological connectedness between the Barbie of 1987 and the sadistic SS officer of the occupation? In my own mind, and no doubt in Parfit's too, these reflections are compounded by doubts, on quite other grounds, about the moral propriety of punishing someone for purely retributive reasons.

This book is supposed, however, to be on *medical* ethics. So what consequences might the line we took on personal identity have for that? Well, one issue in medical ethics that has been receiving a lot of attention recently is that of how one should allocate scarce medical resources. One approach to this issue that is gaining ground in some quarters is based on the concept of a *quality adjusted life year*, or *QALY*.[4] The aim is to try to express the benefits that accrue from various forms of medical intervention in a common unit that takes appropriate account of both the life-extending and the life-enhancing effects of such interventions. The idea is that a year of normal healthy life should count for one unit, but that a year of life that is subject to (health-related) distress or disability should count for less than one, to a degree that reflects the adverse impact of these things on overall quality of life. In these terms, the QALY value of a treatment consists in the difference between the number of QALYs the recipient of the treatment can expect with and those he or she can expect without the treatment in question. Life-extending treatments the effect of which is solely to increase life expectancy thus have a QALY value equal to the extra number of (expected) years of life conferred. Life-enhancing treatments that do not affect life expectancy have a QALY value equal to life expectancy multiplied by the extra value that, owing to the treatment, now attaches to each year. Thus, if a hip replacement operation increases the value of each year of life, of someone with an unaltered life expectancy of sixteen years, from 0.7 to 0.95 of a QALY, then it has a QALY value of $0.25 \times 16 = 4$. If, by enabling the person to take more exercise, the operation also *increases* life expectancy from sixteen to eighteen years, with the same average quality of life as before, then the QALY value of the treatment is $4 + (2 \times 0.95) = 5.9$. Advocates of the QALY approach to health care allocation argue that resources available for health care should be so distributed as to maximise the total number of QALYs generated thereby.

Now it has been pointed out, both in the medical and in the philosophical literature, that consistent application of this criterion is likely to result in patterns of distribution of health care that would intuitively strike one as unjust. Take the case of scarce life-saving treatments; renal dialysis is probably the best known example of such a treatment, in the context of our own health service. (Many patients who need it, who will die without it, fail to get dialysed in Britain today.) Suppose, then, that there were two rival candidates for dialysis between whom there was nothing to choose, save that one was suffering from severe arthritis. Suppose further that there was no reason for thinking that the arthritis would in any way adversely affect the likely success of the dialysis in purely clinical terms. Then the principle that we should so act as to maximise QALYs gained implies that we should favour the candidate who is not suffering from arthritis. For extra years of life which are given to that candidate will correspond to a higher QALY value than an equal number of years given to the other. Of course, in the case of *particular* patients, such considerations would provide only the flimsiest basis for assessing the true overall relative quality of their lives, if there is such a thing; but still, it might seem logical to adopt a general *policy* whereby those free from other health problems should be preferred for life-saving treatment, even where these problems did not affect life expectancy with the treatment. Such a policy would strike many people as inherently unfair. For what it amounts to is that the fact that individuals are unfortunate in one respect is to be taken as a reason for visiting further misfortunes upon them. 'It's bad enough having arthritis', the luckless patient might complain, 'but now you're telling me that *because* I have arthritis, you're going to cause me to lose my life as well!' It looks like a case of 'from him who hath not shall be taken away even that which he hath'.

So what has this got to do with identity? Well, consider another charge that has been laid against the QALY approach, for example by John

Harris,[5] that it is objectionably *ageist*, inasmuch as younger people, given that they are likely to have fewer health problems and a higher life expectancy if treated, will also tend to be favoured over older people for life-saving therapies such as dialysis. Now is this unfair or not? Interestingly, there are *prima facie* plausible arguments on both sides. The argument for saying that it is unfair will run parallel to that just cited in relation to the arthritic renal patient. 'Isn't it bad enough', the older patient might protest, 'that I'm old, that I don't have very many more years of life ahead of me anyway, and that I suffer from several of the ills associated with old age. And now you're telling me that because I'm already unfortunate in all these respects, I'm to be robbed even of such life as I *would* otherwise have to look forward to. Shame on you!' The argument for saying that it isn't unfair is the so-called 'fair innings' argument. The older person, so the argument goes, has already, by definition, lived longer than the younger one. Thus, to give the life-saving treatment to the older patient would be inequitable in terms of years of life lived; the younger patient would get hardly any more life to add to the relatively meagre amount he has already had, whereas the older person, who has already had a relatively generous allowance in this respect, will get even more. Note that this argument implies that one should give preference to a younger over an older patient, even where, because of other health problems afflicting the younger patient, there was nothing to choose between them in terms of quality of life or life expectancy. Indeed, assuming a pluralistic system of values which required us to weigh considerations of fairness against considerations of utility, the fair innings argument might lead one to give preference to the younger patient even if the QALY value of the treatment, as administered to the older patient, was somewhat higher.

It is precisely at this point that questions of personal identity enter the picture. Just what one takes the relative force of these two opposing arguments to be (assuming that one is disposed to be moved by considerations of fairness at all), is going to depend crucially on the moral weight one wishes to attach to the fact that the older person is the *same* as all the younger persons who lived the years that collectively make up his or her life. I put it to you that, from the standpoint of someone who believes that personal identity retains its full moral force over the entire stretch of a person's life, the argument designed to show that it *is* unfair to favour the young in the way that the QALY approach appears generally to demand can only seem like a perverse piece of special pleading. The argument implicitly assumes that different person stages, albeit of the same person, can properly be regarded as independent claimants upon health care resources. But considerations of fairness, so the counterargument would run, must be sensitive to a person's life, regarded as a temporal whole: it isn't, after all, person *stages* to whom the demands of fairness apply, but persons.

Suppose, however, that one sides with Parfit in seeing the moral significance that attaches to personal identity as deriving solely from such psychological connections (of memory, intention, personality or whatever) as link the relevant person stages together, and as having a weight that is a function of such connectedness. Then one is likely to see some merit in the argument that favouring the young – in distributing, say, lifesaving treatment – is indeed objectionably discriminatory; which is not to deny that one would still wish to give weight to the opposing argument as well. In one limiting case, where personal identity was thought to carry its full moral force, undiminished by the passage of time, as applied to any pair of stages of the same person, the fair innings argument would, as we have seen, completely dominate, and the opposing argument be regarded as wholly specious. At the opposite limit, where personal identity in relation to past stages was never to be given any weight, and future stages only to the extent that persons contingently, if irrationally, had a special *concern* about future person stages of themselves, it is the fair innings argument that would be dismissed as specious, and the opposing argument would hold sway. Parfit's position, lying as it does between these two extremes, would result in each of the arguments being regarded as having some force, neither sufficient wholly to defeat the other.

All this, of course, is at the level of fairness. But, as I remarked just now, considerations of fairness themselves would presumably have to be balanced in some way against the essentially utilitarian considerations to which the QALY approach appeals. At the level of fairness, however, what taking a Parfitian view of identity might imply in practice is that one gave some weight to relative youth in adjudicating the claims of rival contenders for some life-saving resource, but a weight that was more liable to be defeated by other considerations than if the fair-innings argument was regarded as having unqualified validity. And that might mean that one was more likely to favour an older over a younger patient when utilitarian considerations were already pulling in that direction. It is perhaps worth remarking that, in the case of dialysis, the QALY-based reasons for favouring the young are in one respect rather less strong than in the case of many other life-saving therapies; for the lower life expectancy of the old counts for less when their death frees the resources for others. In terms of total number of years saved, it may make little difference whether the machine has a relatively rapid turnover of older users, or just one longer term, younger user. (In practice, however, it is highly relevant from the standpoint of generating the maximum number of QALYs that a younger person is more likely to be considered eligible for a kidney transplant, both because that will then free the machine for others and because the patient's expected quality of life with a transplant is far higher than on dialysis.)

I turn now to another much-vexed problem in biomedical ethics: that of the moral status of the human embryo or foetus. Two particular manifestations of this problem are the abortion issue and the issue of human embryo research, though what I have to say will have greater direct relevance to the abortion issue. Now the usual starting point, in philosophical discussions of these issues, is that there is something special about (at any rate) normal human beings beyond early infancy: something that distinguishes them from animals of other species, and which makes it especially wrong to kill them or subject them to potentially damaging experiments without their consent. These attributes include self-reflective awareness, rationality, in Aristotle's sense (that is the capacity to do things for reasons, rather than in response merely to arational drives or impulses), and the related ability to form intentions for the more than immediate future, the power of empathising with others, and the power to converse. Whether or not any of these things are exclusive to human beings (which they almost certainly are not), we could probably agree that no other animal known to science possesses them to an extent that renders them remotely comparable, in these respects, to any normal human being beyond early infancy.

Assuming then that it is attributes such as those I have listed – sufficiently many, to a sufficient degree – that give normal human beings their special moral status and claim to protection from potentially injurious treatment, the following question arises. Is it the *actual* possession of these attributes that confers upon human beings this special moral status, or the *potential* for them, whether or not this potential is currently actualised? At this point philosophers have found themselves confronted with a most embarrassing dilemma. Suppose, first, that it is the actual possession of these attributes that counts, morally speaking. Then one need (for these reasons at any rate) have no particular qualms about abortion, much less contraception. But nor need one think that there is, from an intrinsic standpoint, any very serious objection to infanticide either! (I am ignoring, here, the interests of the parents.) For as regards the actual possession of the attributes that ground our special claim, as human beings, to protection, a newborn infant is actually less well endowed than most adult (indeed many newborn) nonhuman mammals. So, ignoring adverse social consequences, and the possible violation of the interests of others, it would seem that it can be no worse painlessly to kill it or humanely but injuriously to experiment on it, than it is to do this to a dog or a rat.

That is, to say the least, rather difficult to swallow. But the consequences of embracing the other horn of the dilemma are equally unappealing. Abortion, infanticide and, where conception has actually occurred, the 'morning after' pill (which works by preventing implantation) will, once again, be essentially on a par with one another but now equally to be condemned as murder (though some moral weight might be attached to the fact that, in the case of an embryo that is killed very soon after conception, the probability that it would in any case have succeeded in developing to the point where it possessed the attributes that render us morally special is substantially less than in the case of a newborn baby that has most of the worst pitfalls behind it). These, to be sure, are conclusions that many people, particularly Roman Catholics, might welcome. But, first, even if one thinks that it is wrong deliberately to terminate a pregnancy, it seems repugnant to common sense that, say, preventing a newly fertilised ovum from implanting should be just as wrong as infanticide (ignoring side-effects). And secondly, it is far from clear that the logic of this position stops at conception. Suppose we have the situation, now common in *in vitro* fertilisation clinics, where sperm and ova have been mixed together in a petri dish with some nutrients. (A wag in one of my classes asked me whether they used Baby Bio!) Then the system as a whole has the potentiality for the coming into being of a normal human person. If potentiality is what counts, it would appear to follow, therefore, that it would be morally wrong to destroy the contents of the dish even *before* conception had occurred (and in such a way as to prevent conception occurring), even if this were the wish of all interested parties. And presumably ordinary methods of conception would have to be similarly condemned. Of course, contraception is something of which Roman Catholics tend in any case to take a dim view. But not on *these* grounds surely.

Is there, then, a way of resolving this dilemma? Is there a philosophically defensible middle position? Well that depends. What we have to ask ourselves, first of all, is why anyone should be disposed to think that the potentiality for such things as rationality, self-reflective awareness and the rest, should generate a moral obligation on anyone not wilfully to prevent this potentiality from being actualised. One reason would be if one thought that beings with these attributes were a good thing to have around, and (other things being equal) the more of them the better. But this, if true, is only an impersonal sort of reason which speaks to an impersonal kind of good. One instantiation of it would be the thesis that people have a positive obligation to become parents. But even if they do, this would not seem a very compelling kind of obligation, and certainly far weaker than the obligation not to commit infanticide. Unless we are prepared to credit possible people with a claim to be brought into existence, there will not, in general, be any individuals, past, present or future, whose moral claims upon us are violated by a deliberate failure to procreate.

One way in which an individual can come to have a claim upon us is if that individual has an interest in our acting in a particular way. (Whether all interests generate even *prima facie* claims, and if not what is special about those that do, are difficult questions which I shall not here address.) By 'interest', I mean that it is *in* that individual's interests that we so act; the interest need not be grounded in any present desire. A necessary and sufficient condition for an individual to have, in this sense, an interest in our acting or not acting in a certain way is that the individual in question stands to *benefit* by our so doing. (Thus, it could be said to be in the interests of a small child that he or she gets a good education, even though there may be no current desires of the child the satisfaction of which would be furthered thereby.)

Returning then to the potentiality for such things as self-reflective awareness, Aristotelian rationality and the like, the most readily comprehensible way in which such a potentiality could generate a claim on others not to interfere with the realisation of this potential is if there is an individual who stands to benefit by its realisation. Since the focus of our interest here is on the foetus itself, rather than on third parties such as its parents, we can narrow it down further. What would generate a claim would be the existence of an individual who stands to benefit by virtue of *itself* coming to possess these attributes. *And this is where identity comes in.* Suppose we are contemplating terminating a pregnancy. The question then is whether there exists now, or will at the time the termination would occur, the very same individual that, were it allowed to develop normally, would in due course possess such attributes as self-reflective awareness, rationality and so forth.

Of course, this is not all that is required. We must also be convinced that these attributes, the ones that mark us off as special within the animal kingdom, actually are of such benefit that wilfully to prevent an individual developing them is to subject that same individual to a very serious loss. I don't quite know how one would argue for this. But I take it that it is something that most of us believe. For my own part, I am very glad that I am a human being and not a dog, say, though in spite of the phrase 'it's a dog's life', I actually think being a dog, in most English households, is a pretty cushy number. I'm quite sure most dogs don't suffer from my anxieties. Nevertheless, the fact that we have the capacities we do – for reflection, planning, understanding of our circumstances, for engaging with others, through our capacity to converse, to emphathise and to embark on shared projects, and the powers of moral and aesthetic awareness – seems to me to give our lives a richness and depth incomparably greater than that of the lives of other animals (in so far as we can fathom them). Even the life of the most intelligent, active and well-cared for dog seems to me vastly impoverished by comparison to that of any normal human being. To that extent I would heartily endorse Mill's famous remark that 'it is better to be a human being dissatisfied than a pig satisfied'.[6]

But we still have the identity question to contend with. However great a benefit all these things may be to their possessors, they cannot, merely in virtue of that, generate an interest or claim unless the being that stands to enjoy these attributes already exists, albeit not yet possessed of them. There is, of course, *something* that comes into existence at conception and which continues to exist throughout the individual's life; and this is a certain human organism. The embryo and foetus both correspond to stages in the development of the organism. If, then, one thought that it was the human organism that could properly be said to possess such attributes as reflective awareness and rationality, and to benefit by them (in some morally relevant sense) – if, indeed, it is a certain human organism that I am referring to when I use the word 'I' – then it would follow that from the moment of conception there existed something that had a powerful interest in not being destroyed.

One thing that Locke saw very clearly, however, was that we are *not* living organisms. In his *Essay* he makes a stipulative distinction between what he calls the *man* (he wouldn't get away with that nowadays) and the *person*. And by 'man' he means precisely what I am calling the living human organism. (It isn't, of course, what 'man' means in ordinary speech, which I take it is something like, adult male human person.) A *person* for Locke is what you and I are essentially for precisely the period during which we exist at all. And Locke saw that it was a clear implication of his account of personal identity that the identity conditions of persons and of men, in his stipulative sense of living human organisms, failed to coincide. Moreover, he is clearly right in so saying, irrespective of what one thinks of Locke's particular theory. If my brain were to be successfully transplanted into the body of a chimpanzee, it would hardly be appropriate to say that what one had, in relation to my previous body, was the *same* living organism, let alone human organism; but surely I, which is to say the person that I necessarily am, would still exist. And then again, with brain death, the person would now normally be thought of as having ceased to exist, at any rate in that body, but so long as respiration, circulation and metabolism were maintained (albeit by artificial means) one would say that the same living organism persisted.

Given that we are not human organisms, it is thus a substantive question whether, at any given stage after conception, there is actually a person there – understanding now by 'person' whatever it is that we essentially are, without commitment to any particular theory of what constitutes personal identity. For, given that it is the *person* who stands to benefit by possession of such attributes as self-consciousness, rationality and so on, it is only when that person has come into existence, that the potentiality of the corresponding organism will generate a claim on others not to destroy it, in virtue of that very person's interests in this potential being realised. And when the person does come into existence is something that could be settled if (a) we had a correct theory of personal identity and (b) knew all the relevant facts. The theory of identity would present us with some specific relation R, such that any two person stages were to be counted as stages of the same person just in case they were R related. The question, say, 'When did I come into existence?' would thus have the schematic answer: 'At the earliest moment at which there existed something that stood in the relation R to me now.' And when that moment was would then itself be a straightforward matter of fact (whether or not it was at all easy to establish in practice).

Putting things that way highlights a point that seems almost invariably to have been overlooked in discussions of the abortion issue. The question is not just whether, at a given stage of pregnancy, there is *a* person in the womb, but whether it is the same person who, if the foetus were allowed to develop sufficiently would then possess the characteristically human capacities that are the putative source of our special claim to protection. Moreover, it could turn out, if Parfit's view were correct, that it *was* the same person, but that all the same, the psychological connection between a foetus in the womb and the subsequent child, at the earliest moment at which it could be said to possess a concept of self, Aristotelian rationality and so forth was so tenuous that any interest the earlier person could be said to have in the realisation of the foetus's developmental potential would be entirely marginal. Its claim not to be aborted would then be correspondingly very weak.

It's at this point that I must come clean about what I think about personal identity and its moral significance, especially as it relates to human embryos and foetuses. First, with one minor qualification, I am strongly inclined to think, as against Parfit, that it really is, after all, identity that matters in these cases, rather than psychological continuity and/or connectedness *per se*. (The minor qualification concerns fission. I agree with Parfit that if I knew that I was going to be subject to an operation that would split my brain in two and transplant one half into another body, it would be rational antecedently to think of the lives of both halves in the way I would normally think of my own future; Parfit makes the useful suggestion that we should distinguish in such cases between identity and what he calls *survival*.[7] Thus what I am really saying is that it is survival that matters.)

Secondly, I disagree with Parfit's claim that there is no more to our persistence over time than the existence of psychological connections between person stages. Parfit's theory clearly represents a considerable advance over Locke's, inasmuch as he quite properly gives weight to other kinds of memory than experiential memory, and other kinds of psychological connectedness than memory. Newborn babies, let alone foetuses, simply do not qualify as persons, for Locke, seeing that a neonate manifestly is not 'a thinking intelligent being, that has reason and reflection, and can consider itself as itself . . . at different times and places'. This high redefinition of 'person' is rapidly gaining ground in some quarters. But it seems to me regrettable. It is not in accord with ordinary usage and has the effect of pre-empting the issue of our persistence over time, so long as this is identified with the problem of *personal* identity. With a suitable broadening of the concept of memory, so as to encompass any kind of learning, there will be no reason to insist *a priori* that a newborn baby cannot be the same person as some later child or adult, in any ordinary sense of 'person'.

But I would argue that there is, in any case, something wrong with the idea that personal identity can be taken simply to consist in such connections and continuities as are exhibited in consciousness and behaviour. Intuitively, one's identity over time is, I would suggest, conceived of as a *deep* fact: something we think of as lying behind these connections and continuities, something of which the latter are merely a manifestation. It is this feature of our common-sense concept of personal identity that makes it so natural to believe in the soul, though I don't think that our concept of identity is logically committed to any such notion. What is really happening here, it seems to me, is that personal identity is functioning as a *natural kind* concept. Following Mackie,[8] one might draw an analogy with the way in which, according to Kripke,[9] the concept of 'gold' functions. Kripke argues, very persuasively, that the question what makes gold gold is to be understood as a question about *real essence* in Locke's sense.[10] It is, he urges, a mistake to suppose that one could state logically necessary and sufficient conditions for a lump of stuff to be gold, simply in terms of such superficial attributes as colour, malleability, ability to resist certain acids, electrical conductivity and so on. The essence of gold consists not in such attributes as these, but rather in whatever it is about gold that causally sustains and provides the deep explanation for the various superficial attributes by which gold is normally recognised as such. In just the same way, I think it's a mistake to try to *define* identity in terms of psychological connections and continuities. What our identity actually consists in, I suggest, is, once again, whatever, as a matter of scientific or metaphysical fact, normally underlies these more superficial continuities and connections and provides the deep explanation for them. And from a purely secular standpoint, I should have thought that the overwhelmingly most-favoured candidate was a continuity of organisation within those parts of our brain that directly sustain those activities we think of as mental. This would be parallel to saying that what something's being made of gold actually consists in is its being composed of atoms with atomic number 79. We say that because, in the light of modern scientific knowledge, we know that it is this fundamental truth about the nature of gold that explains why, under normal conditions, gold exhibits the density, malleability, chemical, light-reflective and conductive properties that it does.

To repeat, it is, on this view, a largely empirical question what our identity actually consists in, just as it was an empirical question what made gold gold. We do not know precisely what it is about the brain (always assuming that it *is* something about the brain) that serves to sustain manifest behavioural and psychological connections and continuities, and which accordingly grounds our identity over time. But then it is largely mysterious how the brain sustains mental functioning in the first place, and wholly mysterious why some brain functions should be associated with consciousness (the very existence of which strikes me as a complete enigma from the standpoint of physical science). It would seem, however, overwhelmingly probable that these things will turn out to have a *common* explanation: that to understand how the brain sustains mind at all is *ipso facto* to understand what it is for it, so to speak, to sustain the existence of the same mind. At such time, then, as the brain has matured to the point of being able to sustain any characteristically mental functions, I would expect to find in place the neurophysiological substrate of such psychological connections and continuities as are to be found in consciousness and the behaviour we take to manifest mentality. (Even if meaningful, it is hardly plausible that the earliest actions and experiences should be causally and functionally disjoint, like unthreaded beads.) There is, to be sure, no *logical* necessity that the first dawnings of action and awareness (in the womb presumably) should stand in such a relation to the doings and experiences of the adult that they could, on my view, be counted the actions and experiences of the same person. (For example, mind might briefly flower in one part of the brain, only to be extinguished and then develop independently in another part.) But it is surely the most plausible assumption that they do so stand.

What follows from all this, morally speaking, supposing that I am right? Well one thing that follows is that, as regards the abortion issue, it really may make a big difference whether what is being proposed is a late or an early abortion. Clifford Grobstein,[11] who has surveyed the evidence on foetal brain and behavioural development, has concluded that one can confidently rule out the existence of sentience in a foetus of eight weeks or less after conception (which corresponds to what is normally thought of as the first ten weeks of pregnancy). Before that time, if Grobstein has interpreted the evidence correctly, I would argue that early abortion ought to be regarded as morally permissible *tout court*, and that the law probably ought to reflect this, by allowing such abortions on demand. The logic of my argument clearly implies, however, that the late abortion of a perfectly normal foetus is *prima facie* morally wrong.

I shall not here go into the question of what other moral considerations should be thought capable of overriding that *prima facie* wrongness, nor what the law should be, save to make one remark. It does not follow, even if my argument is accepted, that destroying a foetus, at a late stage in its development, or a newborn baby come to that (I see no grounds for regarding the in the womb/out of the womb distinction as having any intrinsic moral significance), is morally completely on a par with killing a child (beyond early infancy) or an adult. The argument for not killing it is that it has, in virtue of its potential for the kinds of things that go to give a normal human life its special worth, a powerful interest in not being killed. And, save that the potential is then actualised, this reason applies to the adult too. But there is another reason why it is so wrong deliberately to end the life of an adult or child beyond early infancy, that does not apply to the foetus or newborn baby. An adult characteristically has a powerful *desire* to go on living; moreover an adult generally has a host of goals, desires, ambitions, projects, for the satisfaction or fulfilment of which continued life is a necessary condition. Death, for the adult, means that many (if not most) of one's hopes and dreams are automatically dashed. In these terms it makes good sense that, if faced with the choice, a doctor should save the expectant mother, in preference to the child she is carrying, assuming that that is the mother's wish; and in general it is perhaps right that the *prima facie* claim to protection of the late foetus and even the newly born, should be susceptible of being more easily overridden in the light of countervailing considerations than that of a normal human being beyond early infancy.

And finally, what of our elderly contender for dialysis? Well, I fear that my view implies that the fair innings argument is fully valid, at the level of fairness. In the passage to old age we never really succeed in placing a moral distance between our present and our earlier selves, however much we may like to believe that we do. And as for Barbie and their like, if this means that they never escape the sins of their youth, it also means that forgiveness is possible; for it means that those who committed those sins are, in a morally relevant sense, still there to be forgiven.

ACKNOWLEDGEMENT

Parts of this article have been published previously in the journal *Bioethics* and are included by kind permission of the editor.

NOTES

1 John Locke (1690) *An Essay Concerning Human Understanding*. A. D. Woozley (ed.) (1964). London: Fontana/Collins, Book II, ch. 31, para. 9, pp. 211–12.
2 Thomas Reid (1941) 'Of memory' in A. D. Woozley (ed.) *Essays on the Intellectual Powers of Man (1785)* London: Macmillan. The relevant chapter, 'Of Mr Locke's account of our personal identity', is reprinted in John Perry (ed.) (1975) *Personal Identity*. Berkeley, CA: University of California Press, pp. 113–18.
3 Derek Parfit (1984) *Reasons and Persons*. Oxford University Press, part III.
4 Alan Williams (1985) 'The value of QALYs', *Health and Social Service Journal*, July, pp. 3–5.
5 John Harris (1986) 'Rationing life: quality or justice?' (unpublished), paper presented to the British Medical Association Annual Scientific Meeting, Oxford 10–12 April, pp. 7–8.
6 John Stuart Mill, *Utilitarianism* in James M. Smith and Ernest Sosa (eds.) (1969) *Mill's Utilitarianism*. Belmont, CA: Wadsworth, p. 39.
7 Derek Parfit (1971) 'Personal identity', *Philosophical Review*, reprinted in J. Perry (1979) *Personal Identity*. Berkeley, CA: University of California Press, pp. 199–223.
8 J. L. Mackie (1976) *Problems from Locke*. Oxford University Press, pp. 199–203.
9 S. Kripke (1980) *Naming and Necessity*. Oxford: Basil Blackwell, pp. 116–44 (original version published 1972).
10 John Locke (1690) *An Essay Concerning Human Understanding*. A. D. Woozley (ed.) (1964). London: Fontana/Collins, Book II, ch. 31, paras. 6–14, pp. 237–42.
11 Clifford Grobstein (1981) *From Chance to Purpose*. Reading, MA: Addison-Wesley, ch. 5.

7   The virtues in a professional setting

William F. May

The Benthamites, observed Melville, would never have urged Lord Nelson to risk his life on the bridge of his ship. The loss of so brilliant a tactician wouldn't have looked good on a cost/benefit analysis sheet. From the British perspective, his heroism would not have produced the greatest balance of good over evil.

Melville's comment slyly suggests that the field of ethics does not reduce to the utilitarian concern for *producing* good. Ethics must deal with *being good as* well as *producing* good, with virtues as well as principles of action. This chapter will explore some of the virtues central to professionals and to those upon whom they practise.

Let it be conceded at the outset that virtue theory is not the whole of ethics. Moralists should not concentrate exclusively on the subject of professional virtue. The terrain of professional ethics covers at least four major areas:

Quandary or case-oriented ethics

The quandarist searches for rules and principles that function as guidelines helpful to the decision maker in resolving moral binds. Some have called this approach dilemmatic or problematic ethics, or, alternatively, ethics for the decision maker. One hopes to arrive at principles that will establish priorities between conflicting goods and evils, rights and wrongs. This dilemmatic approach has dominated the field of professional ethics partly because of its intrinsic prestige in philosophical and theological circles, but partly because of its cultural convenience. The mass media already focus attention on headliner quandaries (whether or not to pull the plug on the comatose patient); and professional education largely organises itself around case study. Students in medical, business, and law schools already attend to cases for much of their professional training. What more natural way to recommend professional ethics as a subject than to adopt the case method in highlighting moral quandaries that a purely technical professional education does not help one resolve?

The moral criticism of systems, institutions, and structures

Quandary ethics alone emphasises too much the perplexities which the individual practitioner faces. It does not examine critically the social institutions that generate professional services, the reward systems that shape professional practice, the complexities of inter-professional and inter-institutional relations, and the delivery systems that allow some problems to surface as cases and others not. On the whole, liberals and radicals have been more motivated than conservatives to raise these structural questions; and social scientists and political theorists better equipped to explore them than conventionally trained ethicists.

Professional regulation and self-discipline

The problem of defective or unethical performance preoccupies the lay person, more than the professional, either the professional practitioner or the professional ethicist. Practitioners only reluctantly accept responsibility for a colleague's behaviour. They do not think of themselves as their colleague's keeper. Ethicists do not find the issue of professional self-discipline intellectually interesting at the level of a quandary. The bad apple is a bad apple. But the neglect of the subject is morally and intellectually regrettable. Professionals wield enormous power, and their reluctance to discipline the bad performer raises interesting moral issues that span the relations between institutions, ethos and virtue.

The subject of virtue

While virtue theory may not deserve pre-eminence of place, it constitutes an important part of the total terrain. Unfortunately, contemporary moralists, with some recent exceptions, have not been too interested in the clarification and cultivation of those virtues upon which the health of personal and social life depends. Reflection in this area is likely to seem rather subjective, elusive, or spongy ('I wish my physician were more personal'), as compared with the critical study of decisions and structures.

Especially today, attention must be paid to the question of professional virtue. The growth of large-scale organisations has increased the need. While the growth of bureaucracies has increased the opportunities for monitoring performance (and therefore would appear to lessen the need for virtue), bureaucracies have also made the society increasingly hostage to the virtue of the professionals who work for them. Huge organisations wield enormous power with which to cover the mistakes of their employees and the opportunity for increased specialisation which they provide, means that few other people – whether lay or professional – know what any given expert is up to. The professional had better be virtuous. Few others may know enough to discredit him. The knowledge explosion is also an ignorance explosion (even the knowledgeable expert is ignorant and dependent in much). If knowledge is power, then ignorance is powerlessness and although institutions can devise mechanisms that limit the opportunities for the abuse of specialised knowledge, ultimately we need virtues in those who wield power. One test of character and virtue is whether a person is virtuous when no one else is watching and a society that rests on expertise needs more people who can pass that test.

I will begin with some general definitions of virtue and then discuss a range of virtues, particularly those pertinent to the so-called helping professions.

A principle-oriented definition of virtue

A moral theory oriented to principles does not altogether ignore the question of virtue, rather it tends to subordinate the virtues to principles. Beauchamp and Childress (1979: p. 235) give the following definition (authors' italics): 'virtues are settled habits and dispositions *to do what we ought to do* (where ought judgments encompass both ordinary duties and ideals)'. This definition subordinates virtues to principles, agents to acts: that is, the question of one's *being* to one's *doing*. It systematically correlates *specific virtues* with specific rules and ideals. Thus the virtue of benevolence correlates with the principle of beneficence, non-malevolence with non-malfeasance, respect with autonomy and fairness with justice.

But the virtues are not simply correlates of principles and rules. They also supply those human strengths, that men and women need precisely at those times when they dispute over principles and ideals. In professional settings, where the arguments sometimes grow fierce, we need, to be sure, modes of reasoning and social mechanisms for resolving disagreements. But philosophical sophistication in the debates between Mill vs. Kant and Nozick vs. Rawls does not necessarily resolve the disputes among us. Sometimes, the philosophers merely transpose the dispute to a more elegant level of discourse. In nineteenth-century England, a fierce quarrel once broke out between two women shouting at one another from second storey windows on opposites sides of the street. An Anglican bishop, passing by with friends, predicted, 'These women can't possibly agree; they are arguing from opposite premises.' In ethics, for similar reasons, the debates rage on.

Just as important as principles may be those virtues that we bring to a dispute: a measure of charity and good faith in dealing with an opponent, a good dose of caution in heeding a friend who approves only too quickly what we think and say, humility before the powers we wield for good or for ill, the discipline to seek wisdom rather than to show off by scoring points, sufficient integrity not to pretend to more certainty than we have, and enough bravery to act even in the midst of uncertainty. Even with the best of theories and procedures, the moral life only too often pushes us out into open terrain, where we must think and act virtuously.

Further a theory of the virtues which merely correlates them with principles fails sufficiently to deal with a range of moral life that does not conveniently organise itself into deeds that we can *perform*, issues about which we can make *decisions* or problems that we can *solve*.

At the close of a lecture that T. S. Eliot once gave on a serious moral issue before an American academic audience, an undergraduate rose to ask him urgently, 'Mr Eliot, what are we going to do about the problem you have discussed?' Mr Eliot replied, in effect, in his no-nonsense way, 'You must understand that we face two different types of problems in life. In dealing with the first kind of problem, we may appropriately ask the question, "what are we going to do about it?" But for another range of human problems the only fitting question is not "what are we going to do about it?" but "how does one behave toward it?"' The first kind of question presses for relatively technical and pragmatic responses to problems that admit of solution; the second recognises a deeper range of challenges – hardy perennials – which no particular policy, strategy or behaviour will dissolve. These problems require behaviour that is deeply fitting, decorous, appropriate. Most of the deeper problems in life fall into this category: the conflict between the generations, the intricacy of overtures between the sexes, the mystery of birth, the ordeal of fading powers and death. 'I could do nothing about the death of my husband', a college president's wife once said to me. 'The only question put to me was whether I could rise to the occasion.' The humanities, at their best, address such questions and less through the deliverances of technical philosophy than through historical narrative, poetry, drama, art and fiction. In the medical profession, the dividing line between Eliot's two types of questions falls roughly between the more glamorous systems of cure and the humbler action of care.

Both kinds of moral challenge call for virtue. But in the second instance, virtues supply us not merely with settled habits and dispositions to *do* what we ought to *do* but also to *be* what we ought to *be*. Virtues come into focus that do not tidily correlate with principles of action: courage, lucidity, prudence, discretion and temperance. Under these challenges we are not simply agents producing deeds but, in part, authors and co-authors of our very being.

None of this self-definition comes easy. Virtues must contend with adversity – not simply the objective adversity of conflict between principles and ideals to which I have already referred but also the subjective adversity of the temptations, distractions, and aversions we must face. Virtues thus do not simply indicate those habits whereby we transform our world through deeds but also those specific strengths that partly grow out of adversity and sustain us in the midst of it.

A virtue-oriented theory of virtue

Alasdair MacIntyre (1981: p. 178) offers a useful start on this second way of interpreting the virtues: 'A virtue is an acquired human quality the possession and exercise of which tends to enable us to achieve those goods which are internal to practices and the lack of which effectively prevents us from achieving any such goods.'[2]

The definition emphasises two important points:

(1) Virtue is an *acquired* human quality rather than an inherited temperament. The two should not be confused. Our annoyance with some people results from their inherited psychic makeup but we confuse their grating temperament with objectionable character.

(2) We should prize the virtues primarily because they make possible the goods *internal* to practices rather than those goods that flow *externally* and secondarily from practices. The virtues make possible the intrinsic goods of studying rather than the *rewards* or results that flow externally from studying such as grades, job, etc.

The role of *public virtue* in the thought of the American Revolutionaries makes clear this distinction between external and internal good. Next to liberty, the Revolutionary thinkers invoked the term 'public virtue' most often in their rhetoric. They defined public virtue as a readiness to sacrifice personal want and interest to the public good. Such virtue, of course, had a kind of utilitarian significance at the level of external outcome. Public virtue, that is, a readiness to make personal sacrifices, was indispensable to winning the Revolutionary War. But if public virtue had only an instrumental value, then the Revolutionaries should have been pleased enough to see the virtue vanish once the war was won. The justification of the practice would lie in the results alone. The Revolutionaries, however, prized public virtue as an *internal* good characteristic of a republican nation. Public virtue belonged to the very *soul* of a republic apart from which it could not be itself, it supplies the glue that holds a republic together. The Revolutionary thinkers quite self-consciously followed Montesquieu: (*The Spirit of the Laws, Book III*). A despotic Government rules by fear; a monarchy governs by the aristocratic aspiration to *excellence*; but a republic, which cannot rely on *fear* or on an aristocratic code of honour, must depend upon public virtue to create a public realm, to be a *res publica*.

Further, if the good that it produces and not the good that it is, alone justifies a virtue, then one might be content with counterfeits or illusions of virtue if these simulacra could get the job done. A Benthamite, for instance, might be tempted to use a Nelson look-a-like on the bridge both to reap the benefit of an inspiring example and to insure the continuing services of a brilliant tactician.

Utilitarians attend so exclusively to results that they see no good in the noble deed *per se* – independent of the good it produces. Thus Mill (ch. 2, p. 22) wrote, 'The Utilitarian morality does recognise in human beings the power of sacrificing their own greatest good for the good of others. It only refuses to admit that the sacrifice is itself a good.' Once dismissing goods *internal* to practice, utilitarians less noble than Mill find it easy not just to instrumentalise but to *corrupt* practice for the sake of outcome.

Not that a virtue-oriented theory of virtue entirely escapes its own set of difficulties when it neglects the question of principles. The question, what should I do, should not completely collapse into the question, who shall I be, and this for at least four reasons: *first*, many virtues *do* correlate with principles and ideas. Without clarification of a *principle* of gratitude it would be difficult to distinguish gratefulness from mere obsequiousness (not an insignificant issue for court life in the eighteenth century, and office life in the twentieth century). *Secondly*, without some common commitment to *principles* of justice, candour etc., it would be impossible to construct a society in which specific configurations of the virtues might flourish.

Thirdly, an exclusive preoccupation with the question, *who* am I, and an indifference to the question, what *ought* I to do – is excessively narcissistic, perhaps even adolescent. The external world quickly fades into theatrical background for one's own expressive acts on centre stage. Max Weber distinguished between value-expressive and goal-oriented actions. Value-expressive acts become more self-expressive than valuable if they do not reckon seriously with the question of what shall I do, and answer that question in the light of principles under which we commonly stand. Thus, I prefer to say that the moral life is a question of being good, *as well as* (and not rather than) doing good.

Finally, MacIntyre is gloomy about the possibility of practising the virtues at all in the large-scale organisation since the bureaucracy, perforce, orients to results, external outcomes, while the virtues evince those goods alone *internal* to practice. I don't deny the existence of tension between the two sorts of goods, especially in a large institutional setting, and the potential compromise in favour of outcomes alone. Efficiency in producing outcomes can overrule all else, yet some large-scale organisations do exist that have not abjectly surrendered everything to the bottom line but have rather signalled their independent and continuing commitment to the internal goods of the practices which they support and organise.

The link between virtues and ideals

Some commentators distinguish between moral rules and moral ideals. They deem rules mandatory and ideals optional, and group character and virtues with the latter. This move runs the danger of reducing character and virtue essentially to the order of the aesthetic.

A word needs to be said here on behalf of the imperativeness of ideals. Just because an ideal looms beyond our reach in the sense that we can seldom directly realise it does not diminish it to the merely optional. One may live under a double responsibility – both to respect the ideal but also to respect the unavoidable difficulties of its realisation in an imperfect world. But this double responsibility does not slacken the ideal to the merely elective. One lives under the *imperative* to *approximate* the ideal: a task which is not merely optional. For example, one may only rarely be able to realise Jesus' command to love one's enemies, but still live under the obligation to approximate this law of perfect love in a very imperfect and violent world. So Niebuhr saw the issue in his debate with the pacifists in World War Two.

Further, the reduction of an ideal to the merely optional neglects an important feature of moral ordeals. Helen Fetherstone – mother, and author of a book about the care of a retarded child – reports that the birth of her child made her feel a little like a person facing the decision to save a drowning person. So to expend your life may be heroic, but the challenge hardly seems optional. You come out of the event a different sort of person from the way you went in. The challenge confronts you at the core of your being and not at some outermost reach of your life where much seems merely optional. Most ideals impinge upon us as something more than optional even while we can only approximate them. Here I stand, I can do no other.

Religion and the virtues

The virtues reflect not only commitments to principles and ideals but also to narratives, the exemplary lives of others, human and divine. Much of the moral life mediates itself from person to person and from communities to persons. As the saying goes, virtues are caught as much as they are taught. The influential narratives, moreover, may be records of divine action, not simply accounts of exemplary human conduct.

At this point, I should concede that philosophers and theologians generally differ in their assessments of the place of religious narratives (mythic and ritual) in the moral life.

Philosophers sympathetic to religious traditions often hold that religious narratives, at their best *illustrate* moral principles. Jesus' sacrificial life, for example, illustrates the principle of beneficence. Kant typified this approach when he held that the really thoughtful person could ultimately dispense with the inspiring example and respond directly to the principle. Thus religion, at the most and at its best, is *morality* for the people: it offers principles heightened and warmed up by inspiring examples.

Religious thinkers, on the other hand, tend to hold that sacred narratives about God's actions and deeds do not merely illustrate moral principles derived from elsewhere. Rather, these decisive events open up a disclosive horizon from which the believer derives the commands, rules, virtues and principles that governs his or her life.

The rabbis, for example, emphasise that the Bible includes two kinds of material, narrative and imperative (*agada* and *halacha*). Christian theologians have argued further that the narrative materials provide the disclosive foundation for the imperatives. For example, the Scriptures of Israel urge the farmer, in harvesting, not to pick his crops too clean but to leave some for the sojourner, for 'you were once sojourners in Egypt'. Thus God's own actions, his care for Israel while a stranger in Egypt, measure Israel's treatment of the stranger in her midst. Similarly, the New Testament reads, 'Herein is love: not that we loved God but that God first loved us. So we ought to love one another.' The imperative derives from the disclosive religious event.

But do these particular scriptural passages simply illustrate and reinforce a more general principle of beneficence, in which case biblical religion, at least in this instance, folds into moral philosophy? A close look at the passage makes it clear that the narrative pushes the believer toward a different notion of love than the philosopher's virtue of benevolence. The general principle of beneficence presupposes the structural relationship of *benefactor* to *beneficiary*, of giver to receiver. How shall I act so as to construct a better future for others? But these scriptural passages put human giving in the context of a primordial receiving. Love others as God loved you while yet a stranger. Thus the virtue in question is not self-derived benevolence but a *responsive love* that impels the receiver reflexively beyond the ordinary circle of family and friendship. The scriptural notion of service differs in source and substance from modern philosophical notions of benevolent or philanthropic love.

The second part of this chapter turns from general definitions to the specific virtues in a professional setting. I will not, however, claim to be talking restrictively about the professional's virtues, as though professionals display a distinctive set of virtues beyond the reach of others. Along that road lies a claim to uniqueness – a gnostic pretension to superiority in knowledge and virtue that swiftly corrupts into high-handedness, condescension and even lawlessness. This essay settles for much less – simply a discussion of the virtues in a professional setting.

It may be useful to begin with the virtues that figure in the debate over the quandary of truth-telling in medicine. That point of departure lets us begin with the role of the virtues in a principle-oriented theory of ethics but then move beyond it.

Often the debate over truth-telling in medicine turns on contending views of the truth's impact on the patient's welfare. Shall I tell the patient the truth and run the risk of frightening him so badly as to interfere with a successful operation? Or shall I avoid telling him the facts in order to protect him? In the latter case, he also suffers. I and others encircle the patient with silence. I subject him to a kind of premature burial. When the debate over truth-telling unfolds in this way, both parties presuppose the same disposition of character and virtue: *benevolence* or, more intensively, compassion. They differ merely on how one makes good on this attitude in truly beneficent action directed to the patient's good or welfare.

The argument, however, can take a second form. The first party again urges the therapeutic lie compassionately intending the patient's good. But this time, the advocates for categorical, or, at least, *prima facie*, truth-telling cite the patient's rights, rather than his welfare. The caretaker owes the patient the truth as a rational creature. The patient is abused if he is managed with something other than candour. The blunt truth may, to be sure, harm the patient, but a lie, in the nature of the case, wrongs him; it subverts his dignity. It subjects the seriously ill patient to a fatal condescension. Thus, two different principles contend in the debate: the patient's welfare vs. the patient's rights; and, correspondingly, two different virtues come to the fore: benevolence vs. *honesty and respect*.

Debate over the issue of truth-telling, of course, can be joined at a very different level, especially when professionals offer informal advice *en famille*. In this variant, pro-truth-tellers argue that honesty is the best policy because the physician becomes vulnerable to lawsuits – if she does not inform patients fully of the risks that surgery entails or if she does not allow a dying man or woman to make appropriate financial arrangements.

Opponents of truth-telling counter that it is easier to manage a dying patient by illusive hope. Both sides decide the issue straightforwardly on the basis of the interests of the staff rather than the patient. Suddenly the virtues of benevolence and honesty vanish and the self-protection of the professional becomes decisive. On the surface, the objective choices would appear to be the same – to tell or not to tell the truth – and yet the virtue or lack of it with which the professional delivers the truth to the patient can alter for the latter its impact and meaning. A very different human environment surrounds a patient when the virtues of benevolence or honesty operate in truth-telling rather than the grubby motives of self-protection alone.

So far, I have discussed the virtues simply as subjective correlates to objective moral principles/obligations. Benevolence correlates with beneficence. Candour correlates with the principle of autonomy. But the subject has already begun to become more complicated. The virtues with which the professional dispenses the truth may condition the very reality he or she offers the patient. This complication displays itself most fully in the link between the truth and yet another virtue, i.e. *fidelity*.

The philosopher J. L. Austin drew the distinction, now famous, between two different kinds of utterances: descriptive and performative. Ordinary declarative or descriptive sentences report a given item in the world. (It is raining. The tumor is malignant. The crisis is past.) Performative declarations do not merely describe the world, but *alter* the world of the person to whom one delivers the declaration. Promises are such performative utterances. (I, John, take thee, Mary.) The promise introduces an ingredient into the world of the hearer that would not be there apart from the vow. As a performative occasion, the marriage ceremony appropriately wastes no time on romantic declarations of love with Wagnerian trombones in the background. The ceremony functions to change the world for two people; it concentrates sparingly on an exchange of vows.

The professional relationship, though less comprehensive and intimate than marriage, is similarly promissory and fiduciary. Taking a client implies a promise to help a distressed person within the limits of one's professional resources. To that degree, the promise alters the world of the patient/client. Correspondingly, to go back on a professional promise is world-altering. That is why the conditions under which a professional can withdraw from a case must be carefully limited.

The distinction between descriptive and performative speech expands the question of the truth in professional life. The talented lawyer, in an important way, alters the world of his troubled client when he tells him performatively that he will take his case. The doctor not only tells descriptive truths, he also makes or implies promises. (I will see you next Tuesday. Or, despite the fact that I cannot cure you, there are other things we can do. I will not abandon you.) The moral question for the professional becomes not simply a question of telling truths, but of *being true to his promises*. Conversely, the total situation for the patient includes not only his disease but also whether others ditch him or stand by him in extremity. (In the background of this expanded sense of the truth lies the scriptural sense of the statement, God can be trusted. He keeps his promises, his covenants, if you will. He is a being-true.)

The fidelity of the professional *per se* will not eliminate the disease or the crime, but it can affect mightily the context in which the trouble runs its course. Thus the virtue of fidelity begins to affect the resolution of the dilemma itself. Perhaps more patients and clients would accept the descriptive truth if they experienced the performative truth. The anxieties of patients in terminal illness compound because they fear that professionals will abandon them. Perhaps also patients would be more inclined to believe in the doctor's *performative* utterances if they were not handed false diagnoses and prognoses. That is why a cautiously wise medieval physician once advised his colleagues, 'Promise only fidelity!'

Truth-telling also involves the virtue of *prudence* and its social specification as *discretion*. Moralists oriented to quandaries tend to concentrate on the question of *whether* one ought to tell the truth. The practitioner knows, or learns painfully, that an equally important question is *how* you tell it – directly or indirectly, personally or with a sparing impersonality. The theologian, Karl Barth, once observed that Job's friends were metaphysically correct in what they had to say about suffering, but existentially false in their timing. They chose a miserable moment to sing their theological arias on the subject of suffering.

Theorists oriented to principles tend to downgrade prudence because they rely on general rules rather than the concrete insight of the practitioner. Correspondingly, the need for prudence shrinks to the adroit crafting of means to ends or the artful packaging of policies. The virtue of *prudence*, to be sure, deals with fitting means to ends. But, as a virtue, it consists of much more than the 'tactical cunning' to which Machiavelli and the modern world diminish the virtue. The medievalists gave a primary place to the cardinal virtue of prudence on the grounds that Being precedes Goodness. An openness to being underlies both being good and producing the good. The marks of prudence include:

(a) *memoria* – being true to the past (rather than retouching, colouring, or falsifying the past);

(b) *docility* – defined as openness to the present, the ability to be still, to be silent, to listen;

(c) *solertia* – readiness for the unexpected.

This essential openness to the past, present, and future fairly summarises what the distressed subject needs from the practitioner in the helping professions.

Prudence demands much more than a facile packaging of what one has to say. Discretion is a question of metaphysical perception, a sense of what the Stoics called the fitting, a discretion that goes deeper than tact, a feel for behaviour that is congruent with reality.

Other virtues deserve attention in any account of professional education and formation and the terms of persisting professional identity. I will conclude by considering a number of these: perseverance, integrity, justice, benevolence and humility.

Perseverance

This is a lowly virtue but indispensable to the acquisition of technical competence under the trying conditions of lengthy professional training today. A young physician once conceded to me that medical school required more stamina than brains. I liked him for saying it. He instantly became my primary care physician because I thought he would have the sense to turn over my case if any complications required a referral. Because that also requires the virtue of modesty.

Perseverance is one of the rather inconspicuous marks of courage. Thomas Aquinas once defined courage as the habit of keeping one's aversions and fears under control. Courage isn't fearlessness, a life free of aversions; it is a matter of keeping one's dislikes, one's laziness, one's fears under control for the sake of the good. It is firmness of soul in the face of adversity. Without such courage, the practitioner fails in that detachment, that disengagement of feelings, indispensable to the delivery of effective service. Most discussions of detachment emphasise the need to disengage one's likes, one's wants, and interests for the sake of a steadfast delivery of services. That goes without saying. But vastly more important, the social worker, the minister, the nurse, and the physician must learn to keep their aversions and frustrations with the client under control.

Integrity

Some thinkers rightly associate this virtue with character itself. Since character is a moral structure rather than a mere temperamental state, one needs a virtue that summarises this inclusive structure, when it is at one with itself.

Integrity draws on the images of uprightness and wholeness. Integrity gets tested at the outset in the forward scramble for admissions to professional schools and in the competition for grades and position. Integrity has to do with moral posture: the upright professional refuses to put his nose to the ground, sniffing out opportunities at the expense of clients and colleagues; he equally refuses to bow before the powerful client or patient, the influential colleague, and outside pressures. Integrity also signifies a wholeness or completeness of character; it does not permit a split between the inner and the outer, between word and deed. As such, it makes possible the fiduciary bond between the professional and the client.

Nothing so demonstrates the indissoluble link between virtue and objective principles and ideals as the virtue of integrity. More than any other virtue, integrity demonstrates that virtue finally pitches the individual out ecstatically beyond himself toward the person, the ideal to which he is committed. We say that a man has lost his integrity when his core identity with those ultimate aims and purposes that ground his life breaks asunder.

Public-spiritedness orients the professional to the common good. The term, 'profession', and the more ancient, though less-often invoked words, 'vocation' and 'calling' have a public ring to them that the terms 'job' and 'career' do not. It ill behooves a professional to sever his calling from all question of the common good and to instrumentalise it to private goals alone. Professionals are often licensed by the state: the society invests in their education; they generate their own public standards of excellence; and they are expected to conform to these standards and to accept responsibility for their enforcement in the guild. Apart from public-spiritedness, the professional degenerates into a careerist and his education becomes a private stock of knowledge to be sold to the highest bidder.

Justice

The notion of the *just* and public-spirited professional suggests more than a minimalist commitment to *commutative* justice, that is, to the fulfilment of duties to others based on contracts. Public-spiritedness suggests a more spacious obligation to *distributive* justice, (above and beyond exchanges through the mechanism of the marketplace). Professionals have a duty to distribute goods and services targeted on basic needs without limiting those services simply to those who have the capacity to pay for them. Some would deny this obligation altogether. Others would argue that the services of the helping professions should be distributed to meet basic human needs, but the obligation so to distribute rests upon the society at large and not on the profession itself. Thus the society, not the legal profession, has the duty to provide services to the poor. This approach argues for a third-party payment system, but the elimination of *pro bono publico* work as a professional obligation.

Still others, myself included, would perceive the obligation to distribute professional services to be both a public and a professional responsibility. Professionals exercise power through public authority. The power they wield and the goods they control are of a public magnitude and scale. Although the state has a primary responsibility for *ministering* justice (an old term for distributive justice), professional groups as well have a ministry, if you will, to perform. When the state alone accepts responsibility for distributive justice, a general sense of obligation diminishes, and the social virtue upon which it depends loses the grounds for its renewal. Professionals need themselves to be actively involved. For example, doctors in the nineteenth century doing such *pro bono publico* work helped to dramatise the need for sanitation laws in our cities.

It should also be noted that such *pro bono publico* work does not merely serve the private happiness of those individuals who receive services, it eventually rebounds to the *common* good and fosters public happiness. Those who receive help are not merely individuals but *parts* of a whole. Thus the whole, in so serving its parts, serves its own public flourishing; it rescues its citizens, mired in their private distress, for a more public life. In the absence of *pro bono publico* work, we signal, in effect, that only those clients who can pay their way into the marketplace have a public identity. To this degree, our public life shrinks; it reduces to those with the money to enter it. Public-spirited professionals not only relieve private distress, they help preserve our common life, in a monetary culture, from a constant source of its perishing.

Benevolence   *> contract tit for tat*

The professional transaction also depends upon a pair of virtues associated with giving and receiving – benevolence (or compassion) and humility. The virtue of benevolent service is the *sine qua non* of the professional relationship. The professional is the giver; the client, receiver. The client depends upon the specialised service that the professional has to offer to meet his needs. The professional, of course, is paid for his or her work, and, like any seller, should be legally accountable for the delivery of goods promised. Compliance with contractual standards is essential; but the legal minimum should hardly be the norm. The professional transaction is giving and receiving, not just buying and selling. Contractualism based on self-interest alone encourages a minimalism, a grudging tit-for-tat – just so much service for so much money and no more. This minimalism is especially unsatisfactory in those professions that deliver help to persons with contingent, unpredictable, future needs that cannot be wholly foreseen in a contract and can only be covered by the habits of service. Benevolence is a pale word for the donative element in the professional relationship; the earlier Western tradition used the stronger words, love and compassion. They bespeak an exposure to the needs of others, beyond calculation, an efficacious suffering with. But our earlier discussion provides ample warning that the virtues of giving should not alone be celebrated. Unqualified and unchecked, they verge on the messianic. They require their counterpart in the virtue appropriate to the role of receiving.

= newan, a student - listenn
+ no confidence

Humility

Humility is not a virtue that one usually associates with professionals. Quite the contrary, long training and specialised knowledge set them apart and touch them with superiority. In popular literature, the professional often takes liberties denied to others as a sign of skill and hard work.

Clearly, the virtue of humility can having nothing to do with obsequiousness, or tentativeness, or ritual expressions of self-doubt over competence. No one needs to see his lawyer nervous before the trial or his surgeon shaky with doubt about his skill. Humility can only be understood as a necessary counterpart to the virtue of benevolence or love.

Idealistic members of the helping professions like to define themselves by giving or serving alone – with others indebted to them. The young professional identifies himself with his competence; he pretends to be a relatively self-sufficient monad, while others appear before him in their distress, exposing to him their illnesses, their crimes, their secrets, or their ignorance, for which the professional as doctor, lawyer, priest or teacher offers remedy.

A reciprocity, however, of giving and receiving, is at work in the professional relationship that needs to be acknowledged. In the profession of teaching, to be sure, the student needs the services of the teacher to assist him in learning but so also the professor needs his students. They provide him with regular occasion and forum to work out what he has to say and to discover his subject afresh through the discipline of sharing it with others. The young rabbi or priest has more than once paused before the door of the sick room, wondering what to say to a member of his congregation, only to discover the dying patient ministering to his own needs. Likewise, the doctor needs her patients. No one can watch the professional nervously approach retirement without realising how much she needs her clients to be herself.

The discipline of receiving is important in still further ways. The professional interview requires addressing but also being addressed, giving, but also taking in; it means both speaking and hearing, the tongue and the ear. The professional's debts, moreover, extend beyond direct obligations to current clients; they also include public monies spent on education, the earlier contributions of clients upon whom he 'practises' while learning his craft, and the research traditions of his profession upon which he daily draws. Humility, finally, is essential to professional self-renewal. No teacher stays alive if he or she does not remain a student. No physician can long dispense a range of professional services if not serviced herself by the research arm of her profession.

Finally, the professional who evinces some of the aforementioned virtues run the danger of taking herself too seriously. Look what it took to get her where she is – stamina, perseverance, courage, integrity, compassion, candour, fidelity, prudence, public-spiritedness and justice. Humility undercuts the temptation to false posturing and heroics. It reminds us of the underground root system of receiving upon which professional life depends.

REFERENCES

Beauchamp, Tom L., and James F. Childress (1979) *Principles of Biomedical Ethics*, First edn. New York: Oxford University Press
MacIntyre, Alasdair (1981) *After Virtue*. Notre Dame, IN: University of Notre Dame Press
Mill, John Stuart (1971) *Mill: Utilitarianism with Critical Essays*, Samuel Gorovitz (ed.). New York: Bobbs-Merrill
Montesquieu, Baron de (1975) *The Spirit of the Laws, Book III*. London: Coller Macmillan

8 Medical ethics, moral philosophy and moral tradition

Thomas H. Murray

The task originally given to me was to discuss 'the philosophical basis of medical ethics'. Without wanting to seem ungracious, I want to argue that medical ethics does indeed have a 'philosophical basis', although not exclusively or even primarily in moral theory. Medical ethics has a basis in philosophy's long and (mostly) honourable tradition of practical ethics – of attempting to think systematically about the moral problems that people actually face. Whether it also has a basis in moral theory is a more perplexing question.

In an effort to understand the relationship between medical ethics and moral philosophy, I will need to explore several issues. The first problem is to describe the currently dominant model of that relationship, deductivism and to examine its shortcomings. Then I will explore the recent resurgence of attention to the tradition of practical reasoning about cases of conscience commonly called casuistry. 'Casuistry', as a concept, has multiple meanings and even more connotations and historical associations. I hope to add some clarity to discussions of casuistry and deductivism by distinguishing between two core meanings of casuistry:

(1) as immersion in the particularity of specific cases or problems coupled with the inescapable need for interpretation; and

(2) as a claim about the relation between moral judgement and moral theory as sources of moral knowledge.

About (1), I will argue that immersion and interpretation are indispensable elements of any competent analysis of cases or problems. Deductivism, in its emphasis on theory, can lead to inadequate attention to the specifics of cases or to a mistrust of interpretation. But these elements of the casuistic method – immersion and interpretation – are also employed by conscientious deductivists. About (2), I hope to begin what must become a more thorough discussion about the sources of reliable moral knowledge and suggest that scholars in medical ethics begin to think more about the concept of moral tradition and attend to recent scholarship on the idea of tradition.

Deductivism and its deficiencies

Most writers on medical ethics or bioethics seem to share a conviction that the correct way to make moral judgements – decisions about specific cases or types of cases – is to proceed deductively: by a progression from moral theory, through intermediate principles, maxims or rules, finally to the judgement itself. We justify our moral judgements in the opposite direction: by appealing to intermediate level principles, maxims or rules, which are justified in turn by the moral theory from which they have been deduced. If this is essentially how moral reasoning proceeds and is justified, then we would be correct to call medical ethics a species of applied moral philosophy, since it would consist in the more-or-less straightforward application of abstract, general moral theories.

The deductivist approach is not confined to any particular moral theory. Rather, it is a way of conceiving the relation between moral judgement and moral theory, and it suggests a particular method for doing medical ethics – proceeding from general theory down to judgements about cases. Deductivists come in many guises: utilitarians (such as Peter Singer);[1] secular Kantians (such as H. Tristram Engelhardt);[2] contractarians (such as Norman Daniels);[3] Protestant Christians (such as Paul Ramsey)[4] and scholars from other religious traditions. Despite their differences over theory and substance, what all deductivists share are interrelated accounts of moral judgement and moral justification and a belief in the primacy of theory. Recent analyses of the relation of ethics to medical ethics, though, have raised doubts about all three elements of the deductivists' position.

Several prominent philosophers have claimed that in the relationship between moral philosophy and medical ethics, moral philosophy has gained the most. In an article provocatively titled 'How medicine saved the life of ethics', Stephen Toulmin argued that 'proper attention to the example of medicine has helped to pave the way for a reintroduction of "objective" standards of good and harm and for a return to methods of practical reasoning about moral issues ...'.[5] Medicine that is, saved ethics from the aridity of excessive abstraction and the 'miasma of subjectivity'.[6] Alasdair MacIntyre in 'What has ethics to learn from medical ethics?' claims that 'at this particular stage of their historical dialogue it is medical ethics that has in the main to be the teacher, ethics the pupil'.[7] MacIntyre bemoans contemporary moral philosophy's 'preoccupation with rules'; as much as devotees of the different theories disagree over the merits of these theories, 'they never seem to doubt that the intellectual content of morality is just such a set of universal rules or that moral judgement consists in the application of such a rule to a particular case'.[8]

The notion that ethical theory has more to gain from its relationship with medical ethics than the other way round is not the common way of conceiving the relationship. Therefore, we should look in more detail at the disadvantages of the deductivist approach. Probably the most often mentioned objection is that since moral theories are generally too abstract to be directly applicable to specific moral judgements, there is a temptation in deductivism to be inattentive to the particularities of cases. Rules can be applied mechanically and insensitively. Another aspect of this inattentiveness is a remoteness from the realities of the clinic leading to a focus on unimportant features of a case while the important aspects go unnoticed.[9] Inattentiveness and remoteness are dangers, but there is an abundance of excellent work in medical ethics by deductivists who overcome temptation and immerse themselves in the lived realities of the situations about which they write.

Other intellectual difficulties with deductivism are not so readily overcome. Most situations are complex enough to invoke more than one fundamental principle; unless you have some definitive scheme for ordering principles, no conclusive answer seems possible. What is more, there will be times when your theory will be too indeterminate to yield an answer. This is particularly disconcerting when it seems to most reasonable and reflective persons that the correct answer is obvious. The embarrassment becomes worse when people's considered judgements are actively opposed to the answer the theory appears to offer.

Apart from these intellectual shortcomings, deductivism suffers from a number of other difficulties. It typically pays little or no attention to the social or historical contexts in which moral problems appear (and moral theories develop); it slides over the sometimes inconvenient fact that human beings must pass through a prolonged period of dependency and arationality before becoming rational moral agents; and it offers a highly dubious account of moral judgement.

In its quest for generalisable rules binding on all persons in all circumstances, deductivism may fail to realise the importance of particular social circumstances, especially the roles people occupy, the relationships in which they participate and the expectations appropriate to both. Annette Baier's recent call for a focus on trust between persons as a fundamental issue in ethics is one manifestation of dissatisfaction with the asocial tendencies of deductivism.[10] MacIntyre criticises the search for an Archimedean moral perspective for its portrayal of the moral agent as having a 'ghostly, abstract and largely disembodied existence'.[11] The moral agent, according to many contemporary moral theories, exists prior to and outside of any social forms. This conception of moral agency is motivated by a desire to find a standpoint for ethics that can transcend the myopia and prejudices of particular cultural moralities. Exposure to a diversity of cultures has convinced many people, including many philosophers, that transcultural, transhistorical abstract principles are the only alternative to a thoroughgoing normative relativism. Whether the program to find an ethic free of cultural and historical grounding is either feasible or necessary is too large a question to address fully here. We can, however, point to the fact that despite the failure of any one theory to be universally persuasive, even mass, pluralistic societies manage to limp along and make moral judgements – a phenomenon deductivists must explain. Something enables cultures to embrace, even if they are not certain how, a set if not a system of shared normative judgements.

Attenuated though they may seem, our moral traditions are lively enough to permit social life to continue. The professions are one place where the genuine vitality of moral traditions may be especially apparent. Toulmin writes: 'we find ourselves born into communities in which the available ways of acting are largely laid out in advance: in which human activity takes on different "forms of life" (of which the professions are one special case), and our obligations are shaped by the requirements of those forms.'[12]

Deductivism is also prone to be unreflective about the moral tradition of which it is a part. The emphasis in secular moral theory, for example, on an ethic of autonomy and liberty ought to be more conscious of its roots in the idea of individualism, and of the historical circumstances in which individualism arose. This sort of historical consciousness will neither establish nor refute an ethic of autonomy, but it will enrich our understanding of its scope and limitations.

When deductivist theories, in their hunger for a universal principle, fix on one that identifies rationality as the essential capacity possessed by moral agents and the subjects of moral concern, they risk ignoring an inescapable fact of human existence: that rational persons begin as profoundly dependent, arational beings. To develop into rational moral agents they must be properly nurtured, taught a conception of the good and given practice in behaving virtuously. A moral theory which has little useful to say about the conditions for the possibility of its own development is seriously incomplete.

A last criticism of deductivist theories is that they provide an unrealistic account of how sound moral judgements are actually made. According to the deductivist model, correct moral judgements are those which conform to the principles under which they are subsumed. If moral deliberation works in a top-down mode (from theory through intermediate principles to judgement) then the starting point – the moral theory – ought to make a considerable difference in where one ends up, and widespread agreement on a variety of cases would imply that people ought to agree at the level of theory as well. The deductivist account must explain, then, the contrary results widely found in the experience of common moral discourse, where people are able to agree about particular judgements without agreeing at all about the supposedly fundamental principles. Perhaps the most notable and best documented instance of this was the work of the US's National Commission for the Protection of Human Subjects of Biomedical and Behavioral Research. Both Toulmin who served on the Commission's staff and Albert R. Jonsen, a bioethicist member of the Commission, report that the Commissioners were able to reach agreement on almost all substantive points by patient attention to the specific cases. Only when they tried to 'justify' their concrete judgements in terms of general moral theories did their deliberations begin to resemble what is said to have occurred during the construction of that tower in Babel.[13]

Toulmin and Jonsen realised that they were participating in a sustained modern example of case-centred reasoning, or casuistry.

Casuistry

In its root meaning, casuistry simply denotes a 'concern with individual cases'.[14] In practice, casuistry involves the close analysis of particular cases, in order to discover what the proper judgement of the case ought to be. English and American common law are casuistic in their method of case analysis. One must find the appropriate precedents for a case, and analyse them to learn where they are relevantly similar and dissimilar. The process is aided by a handful of maxims, rough rules of thumb, for example, *volenti non fit injuria* – with consent, there is no injustice.

Casuistry as a method of practical reasoning in ethics is characteristic of Judaism, where the Law, established in the Pentateuch, had to be interpreted as practical questions arose. The word 'casuistry' has come to have a pejorative connotation through criticisms of one of its ever-present dangers: the possibility that overly subtle distinctions and twisted logic will be used to reach not the right result, but the one desired.

One of the defining characteristics of casuistry is the relative weight it places on immersion in the particularities of the case. This is not, in principle, incompatible with an ultimate reliance on general moral principles. Paul Ramsey, one of the most distinguished Protestant writers on medical ethics, practises a very rigorous form of casuistry in which he combines fierce attention to detail with an equally fierce commitment to theological principles.[15] Ramsey recognises, though, that the movement from principle to case requires interpreting the meaning of the principle for the issues at hand.[16] Ramsey is clear that his principles come directly from his theological commitments, and that he will follow them wherever they lead, even to judgements that challenge a widespread social concordance. His opposition to all non-therapeutic research on children, no matter how innocuous, is an example. For him, the meanings of faithfulness between physician or researcher and patient, and of parental care for children, do not permit research which is not aimed at the child's medical benefit.[17]

The first few brave (or foolish) souls who took their ethical theories into the medical clinic quickly learned two things: first, that practical moral problems were often exceedingly complex and unclear, and that the first step had to be an *immersion* in the particularities of the case specifically, and into the realities of the clinic generally. To mention just one sort of consideration, a would-be ethics consultant had to know something of the expectations of physicians, patients, nurses and family, and whether those expectations were reasonable given the usual practices of the professions and institutional policies as well as the history of the particular case. But the ethicist also had to be able to criticise practices and expectations should they be found to be harmful or to serve ignoble ends. But to criticise such practices intelligently, we need far more than a shallow understanding of them; we need to understand what they are intended to accomplish, whose interests they serve and how well, the common ways in which they malfunction, and the merits of whatever alternatives exist, all of which require a reasonable familiarity with the social and historical contexts in which the problem arises.

A second lesson rapidly learned was that moral theories are not self-applying. Theories, principles, rules or maxims must be *interpreted* in the context of the particular case at hand. Those who would provide ethical advice have to ask what a commitment to autonomy, or dignity, or sacredness or the common good means, for example, in the context of an encounter between a tired physician and an apparently rational but self-destructive patient. There are facts to be considered, ambiguities to be identified and assessed, and, most likely, a variety of considerations to be weighed before a reasonable moral judgment can be made.

Casuistry as immersion and interpretation

Every effort to provide guidance on practical moral problems must necessarily be casuistic in the sense of being case-centred if it is to be at all competent. Making a sound moral judgement requires immersion in the specific facts of the case because it requires interpretation, both of the specifics, for their moral pertinence, and of the principles being applied, as to their meaning in the context of the particular case. Even some of the severest critics of casuistry found themselves, when confronted with actual cases, employing its methods. Martin Luther burned a copy of *Summa Angelica*, a popular work of casuistry in his time, along with the papal bull announcing his excommunication. But he also used a dubiously fine distinction to help an ally in his marital difficulties, and argued elsewhere that certain lies were not sinful when they were done with a good heart for a good cause or for love.[18] Practical reasoning about cases of conscience requires immersion and interpretation no matter how rigorous and ascetic we wish to be.[19]

Interpretation, as an inescapable feature of practical reasoning, is also the source of its greatest temptation. It is inescapable for several reasons. Theories, we have already said, are not self-applying. Indeed, there is a rough trade-off between generality (a distinctive virtue of theories) and applicability: the more generally a theory is stated, and hence the greater its scope of potential application, the more interpretation is required for any particular application.[20]

New circumstances compel new interpretations even though technology can not and should not stand morality on its head. The recent debate over a definition of death is an illustration of what I mean. For centuries, we had lived comfortably with a vague notion about what, precisely, comprised the death of a person. We could wait until the heart ceased beating before people began to do things to the body that would have constituted assault on the living. Two factors contributed to the need for a new interpretation. The mechanical respirator, for one, gave us on occasion the power to sustain a person whose entire brain, including the brainstem, had ceased to function. We had to face the question whether discontinuing the respirator in such circumstances violated our prohibitions against assault or killing. Increasingly successful attempts to transplant organs intensified the need for a clear definition of death. By the time the heart had stopped, those organs which might have been transplanted would have been severely damaged through a lack of oxygen. The wrongness of assault, mutilation, or murder endures; the moral problem is to interpret those prohibitions in light of new circumstances to see if what we mean by 'mutilation', etc. includes removing the kidneys from a person's body in which the entire brain has ceased to function but whose physiological functions are being maintained by a ventilator and other technological means.

Although technology is not the only source of new moral questions, it is the one most often cited. But new social arrangements also create the need for new interpretations. Few would disagree with the claim that children have a moral obligation to ensure that their elderly parents are cared for.

But when a great many elderly are surviving far longer, some with profound disabilities, when offspring are more likely to live a considerable distance from parents, when women as well as men are likely to be employed, when skilled nursing care becomes terribly expensive, in short, when the social circumstances of adult offspring and their aging parents change, the meaning of the moral obligation to care for one's parents must be reinterpreted, not to eviscerate it, but to understand how it might be fulfilled.

The most serious criticism levelled against casuistics is that interpretations may be faulty or self-serving. Without question, interpretation can be done well or poorly, or with greater or lesser impartiality. People can and do engage in logic-chopping and the making of precious distinctions in order to evade moral responsibility for themselves or those whose interests they serve. This is, quite simply, an ever-present danger wherever interpretation is necessary. But to condemn *all* interpretation because it is occasionally misused is foolish. It is foolish because, as Aristotle reminds us, it is a mark of wisdom not to demand any more precision than the subject matter permits. And ethics, like politics, is an inexact science.[21] But we should also note that interpretation is universally required of ethical theories. Thus the first response to the criticism that casuistics is flawed because it relies on interpretation is simply to note that interpretation is inescapable if we are to speak to practical issues at all. Sound, sensitive moral judgement and immersion into the particularity of the case are intrinsic to all forms of sound moral reasoning.

Some proponents of deductivism fear that interpretation will lead inexorably to laxness. They desire to preserve rigour and asceticism by holding interpretations that excuse conduct to a bare minimum. They do so by allowing few distinctions and by minimising the effect particular circumstances will be allowed to have on the interpretation of general prohibitions. The danger in this approach is that in our desire to avoid laxity we will create instead a rigid and legalistic 'tyranny of principles' that tramples not only mercy but also equity.[22] In practice, justice comes not from the inflexible application of moral or legal rules, but from equitable judgements in which rules are interpreted in the light of particular circumstances. What constitutes a 'reasonable' morally sensible interpretation cannot itself be reduced to a precise principle. (Or, at least, no one has yet succeeded in doing so.) Discretion is always necessary: by judges in interpreting the law; by all would-reasonable beings in interpreting the demands of morality. Aristotle grasped this point in his discussion of equity, justice and absolute justice: 'While it is true that equity is just and in some circumstances better than justice, it is not better than absolute justice. All we can say is that it is better than the error which is generated by the unqualified language in which absolute justice must be stated. And equity essentially is just this rectification of the law, where the law has to be amplified because of the general terms in which it has to be couched'.[23]

The inexact science of ethics leaves us always with a tension between the dangers and attractions of ascetic rule-following on the one hand and pliant case-centredness on the other. The former is attractive for its rigour, its stress on generalisability, universality and hence impartiality, its potential use as a critical, reformist force and its neat logicality. We have already mentioned its disadvantages. Casuistics has the advantage of being forthright about the limitations of pure principles, and the need for wise interpretation in the light of particularity. Its flexibility is also its greatest invitation to misuse. Whether casuistics which is not firmly based on moral theory is also irretrievably relativistic is our next topic.

Casuistry and the foundations of moral knowledge

In its first meaning – as sound case-reasoning requiring immersion and interpretation – casuistry is fully compatible with deductivism's belief that moral principles are the primary source of moral knowledge. But a number of the criticisms brought against deductivism cast doubt on that belief and suggest instead that the relationship between moral judgements and moral theories is more complicated. Firm, clear and considered judgements may be at least as sure a source of moral knowledge as our moral theories. Perhaps neither is more 'fundamental' than the other.

There are times when moral judgements are reformed under the insistent force of our efforts to achieve consistency among the many kinds of moral judgements we must make, and our unceasing desire to create concepts and ever-more-abstract generalisations to account for our judgements. But there are also times when principles are altered in response to irresolvable conflict with clear considered moral judgements.

It may be helpful to see the dispute between deductivism and casuistry over the relationship between theory and judgement as being analogous to the difference between mathematics and science. Deductivism, especially in its more formalistic modes, tends to resemble mathematics. It emphasises the creation of formal systems of abstract symbols (or concepts) and the working out of logical interconnections and implications. Applicability is not particularly important; elegance and formal logical coherence are. The principal tests of mathematical theory are *internal*, pertaining to rational consistency; an *external* test, say against empirical observations, has little or no meaning.

Casuistry's account of the relation between theory and external tests, by contrast, more resembles science. In science, theory ultimately is disciplined by its contact with *external* data. Scientific theory should also pass the test of logical consistency, but not at any price. If laboratory data compel us to regard the behaviour of light as sometimes a wave and sometimes a particle, so be it, at least until some new theory comes along that explains the phenomena as well under a single conceptual entity. Scientific theory, then, must face both external and internal tests. The simplistic notion that one confounding observation is enough to topple an established theory was discredited by historians and philosophers of science.[24] But no matter how popular or logically consistent a theory might be, if it repeatedly fails to deal with the data it will ultimately tumble.

I do not mean by this account to portray scientific theory as playing a passive role. This would be close to repeating the errors of inductivist theories of science. Theory does not spring forth from data, nor is it merely a summary of the observations. Scientific theory like all other kinds of theory is the product of creative acts of the human imagination. Furthermore, theories affect the way we see phenomena: they direct our attention towards certain aspects and away from others. They are in this way like maps, picking out highly selected features from a terrain that could be described in uncountable ways.[25] Good scientific theories, like good maps, successfully identify the significant relevant features that will allow us to accomplish the purpose for which they were designed: driving the interstate highways or backpacking in the wilderness; explaining shadow casting or gravitational interactions with light. Admitting considered moral judgements as legitimate candidates for moral knowledge does not condemn us to hopeless subjectivity and moral relativism any more than science's reliance on fallible human observers and always-revisable theories condemns it to the depths of subjectivity and epistemological relativism. That our scientific knowledge can never be certain and perfect, that science is irreducibly a fallible human social activity, that the kind of objectivity we attain is intersubjective agreement, that theory and observation are in continuous dialectical interaction – all these properties of science do not undermine people's faith in scientific knowledge. Yet our moral knowledge, so similar in many respects, is little trusted. In particular, deductivism professes to have little or no faith in the 'data' of ethics – considered moral judgements and moral maxims developed out of the experience of a moral tradition. We must therefore turn to the nature of moral judgements, 'moral tradition', and the potential within moral traditions for dynamism and reform in my final section.

Moral judgement and moral tradition

How do we ever know that a moral judgement is sound? There are a limited number of possibilities. We could subscribe to some form of deductivism, and say that a judgement is sound when it conforms to our moral theory. We could embrace G. E. Moore's notion of 'good' as a simple, non-natural property known to us through intuition. We could join with the emotivists and abandon any claim that moral judgement could mean more than a grunt of approval or distaste. Or we could accept that we stand in a tradition of moral judgements and moral practices that has been in continuous development over millennia, parallel to, but not identical with, traditions in moral theory. A key element of our tradition is self-criticism – the perpetual effort to make sense of judgements and practices by constructing generalisations at ever-higher levels of abstraction. In this account moral theory is in partnership with moral judgement as the two function in concert to construct a coherent set of practices.

MacIntyre is painfully convincing in his portrayal of a culture which has inherited incompatible fragments of moral theory from many traditions.[26] A failure to create universal, substantive moral theories need not mean a parallel failure to establish traditions of practical moral judgement. Despite the existence of certain moral controversies which appear intractable at the moment (abortion, for instance), we seem to have a broad and solid common ground of agreement on many moral issues.

Perhaps moral judgements stand in relation to a moral tradition (including but by no means limited to the systematising efforts of moral philosophers and moral theologians in that tradition) in much the same way that the data of scientific observations stand to scientific theory. If this is so – and much more work would have to be done to buttress the plausibility of this claim – then we can begin to respond to the most severe criticism of casuistics in its second sense (when it claims that moral judgements are a form of moral knowledge). The criticism is that moral judgements can never do more than reflect the prejudices of whatever culture offers the judgements. Morality, then, would indeed be nothing more than an 'ideology' with all the odious connotations attaching to that idea. It would be society's means of excusing itself for its exploitations, and of dampening whatever twinges of conscience might otherwise have arisen.

It is certainly true that particular moral judgements, the 'data' of morality, may be misleading (as can be the data from scientific experiments). But we need not be incurably blind to mistaken judgements. We can detect possible errors in moral judgements in several ways. We notice inconsistencies between moral judgements that, upon careful consideration, appear similar in all relevant respects. Or our attempts to formulate generalisations might reveal other inconsistencies. The patchwork of laws dealing with black slaves in the antebellum south in the US treated them as persons in some respects and children or even non-persons in others.[27] May not a case-centred ethics work similarly?

Another response is to note that the criticism is based on an empirical claim – that without moral theory (as the concept is currently understood) moral reform would be impossible. It would be interesting to put this claim to the test. One approach could be to encourage studies in the history of moral judgements and practices. If, as seems apparent, there have been momentous changes in moral judgements and practices, more for the better than for the worse, it would be helpful to know from where those changes arose. From new ideas? From new interpretations of old ideas? Or did changing practices precede the changing ideas? Studies of this sort may help us to understand whether the temptation to ideology or mere reflection of prejudice is irresistible, or, alternatively, if genuine reform beyond crude self-interest is possible.

We moderns seem to have an impoverished view of a culture's resources for moral change. There is a vast panoply of morally relevant beliefs and practices, any element or combination of which can serve as a spur to reform. Edward Shils describes a number of 'endogenous' and 'exogenous' forces that press traditions, including moral traditions, to accommodate and change.[28] Within mass, pluralistic cultures, there are many such pressures and resources. The common law, for instance, shares many concerns with a society's moral tradition (where they are not one and the same), as do the traditions governing the actions of the various professions. Where there are many moral traditions, they communicate with and affect one another to a greater or lesser degree. There will also be many non-moral beliefs that are none the less highly relevant to morality e.g. beliefs about God, about the nature of persons, or about the nature of the good for persons. And there is always the unceasing dialectical interplay between and among moral theory, moral judgements and the intervening levels of generalisations.

Unfortunately, invoking the idea of moral tradition invites misunderstanding. For many people, it connotes an unresponsive social conservatism, and indeed, a narrow concept of 'tradition' is often used in an effort to bludgeon people into accepting a particular set of beliefs and practices that can be found in the past, and that serve the interests of those pleading for a return to 'traditional' values. In fact, our moral traditions are much richer than that, and can as readily stand in opposition to political conservativism. One recent and important example is the pastoral letter written by the US National Conference of Catholic Bishops on the economy. Entitled *Economic Justice for All: Catholic Social Teaching and the US Economy*, the letter contains stern criticism of capitalism because it permits extensive poverty to exist in the midst of great wealth, and denies many people the opportunity to find dignity through productive labour. The letter's language is often striking. Noting the increase in economic interdependence, the letter asserts these new links 'create hope for a new form of community among all peoples, one built on dignity, solidarity, and justice'.[29] Earlier drafts of the letter so disturbed conservatives that a group of Catholic laypersons formed a 'Commission' of their own to defend capitalism and to criticise governmental social programmes.[30] The pastoral letter and the response it evoked testify to the reforming vitality of moral traditions. Thus living moral traditions will not be so easily claimed by political conservatives as many people fear. Indeed abandoning tradition to one end of the political spectrum may be one of the worst mistakes a culture can make.

Jaroslav Pelikan, from his perspective as a scholar of one particular tradition, Christianity, describes the place of tradition in the humanities with characteristic eloquence: 'The growth of insight – in science, in the arts, in philosophy and theology – has not come through progressively sloughing off more and more of tradition, as though insight would be purest and deepest when it has finally freed itself of the dead past. It simply has not worked that way in the history of the tradition, and it does not work that way now. By including the dead in the circle of discourse, we enrich the quality of the conversation.'[31] This is as true of traditions in practical ethics as it is of other strands of tradition, including the humanities.

We are always acting in concert with, in reaction to, or in ignorance of our traditions. But these same traditions do not condemn us to hopeless stasis or a relativity beyond reason and objective criticism. Within and among our traditions, we have substantial resources for reform. These resources in tradition are more than potent enough to serve as counterweights to that part of the hand of tradition which is self-deceiving or dead.

They will not permit us the Archimedean stance, but that may be a false goal in any event; they very possibly will create a reflective climate in which particular moral judgements can be made with some assurance. This does not condemn us to moral stagnation because we have ample proof of the dynamic power of traditions to change in response to the criticisms they provoke by their own inconsistencies. That proof exists in the conversations carried on at all times in all cultures about moral problems. It thrives at this very moment in many forms not least of which is the tradition of practical medical ethics.

NOTES

1 Helga Kuhse and Peter Singer (1985) *Should the Baby Live: The Problem of Handicapped Infants*. New York: Oxford University Press.

2 H. Tristram Engelhardt (1986) *The Foundations of Bioethics*. New York: Oxford University Press.

3 Norman Daniels (1985) *Just Health Care*. New York: Cambridge University Press.

4 Paul Ramsey (1970) *The Patient as Person*. New Haven, CT: Yale University Press.

4 Stephen Toulmin (1982) 'How medicine saved the life of ethics', *Perspectives in Biology and Medicine* 25 (4) p. 740.

6 *Ibid.*, p. 41.

7 Alasdair MacIntyre (1978) 'What has ethics to learn from medical ethics?', *Philosophic Exchange* 2 (4) pp. 37–47.

8 *Ibid.*, p. 41.

9 John Arras (1991) 'Getting down to cases: the revival of casuistry in bioethics', *Journal of Medicine and Philosophy*, vol. 16, pp. 29–51.

10 Annette Baier (1986) 'Trust and antitrust', *Ethics* 96 (2) pp. 745–6.

11 Alasdair MacIntyre (1978) 'What has ethics to learn from medical ethics?', *Philosophic Exchange*, 2 (4) p. 41.

12 Stephen Toulmin (1982) 'How medicine saved the life of ethics', *Perspectives in Biology and Medicine* 25 (4) p. 745–6.

13 *Ibid.*, p. 741; Albert R. Jonsen (1986) 'Casuistry and clinical ethics', *Theoretical Medicine*, pp. 65–71.

14 Werner Stark (1973) 'Casuistry', *Dictionary of the History of Ideas*. New York: Scribners.

15 See, e.g., Ramsey (1970) *The Patient as Person*. New Haven, CT: Yale University Press.

16 As an example see his introduction to *The Patient as Person* where he explains the theoretical underpinning of his book: the covenant of faithfulness between physician and patient, as an expression of the covenant of man with man, and God with man.

17 Ramsey's position was first stated in *The Patient as Person*. It was further developed in an exchange with Richard A. McCormick. The pertinent references are: McCormick (1974) 'Proxy consent in the experimental situation', *Perspectives in Biology and Medicine*, 18 (Autumn) 2–20; Ramsey (1976) 'The enforcement of morals: Nontherapeutic research on children', *Hastings Center Report* (August) 21–30; McCormick (1976) 'Experimentation in children: sharing in sociality', *Hastings Center Report* (December) 41–6.

18 Stark (1973) 'Casuistry', *Dictionary of the History of Ideas*, p. 262. New York: Scribners.

19 For an interesting comparison of case-reasoning approaches see Baruch A. Brody, Richard A. McCormick, David H. Smith, and Stephen Toulmin (1981) 'Marriage, morality, and sex-change surgery: four traditions in case ethics', *Hastings Center Report* (August) pp. 8–13.

20 Arthur E. Murphy (1984) *The Theory of Practical Reason*. La Salle, IL:

Open Court, shows how Kant's conception of practical reason with its emphasis on formal rationality and objectivity, misleads us about the place of objectivity in ethics. 'The requirement of objectivity in moral judgement is a requirement *for* the use of normatively cogent procedures in this activity, not the imposition upon it of an imperative which decides by "rational" fiat what in general is to be done and commands our unconditional submission to its dictates'. (p. 293).

21 Aristotle, (1955) *Nichomachean Ethics*. Book II, ch. 3, pp. 27–8. Baltimore MD: Penguin.

22 Stephen Toulmin (1981), 'The tyranny of principles', *Hastings Center Report* (December) pp. 31–9.

23 Aristotle (1955) *Nichomachean Ethics*. Book V, ch. 10, p. 167. Baltimore, MD: Penguin.

24 The best-known study of this and related issues is Thomas S. Kuhn (1962) *The Structure of Scientific Revolutions*. University of Chicago Press.

25 The map metaphor for scientific theory is developed in Stephen Toulmin (1960) *The Philosophy of Science*. New York: Harper Torchbook. See especially ch. 4.

26 Alasdair MacIntyre (1981) *After Virtue*. Notre Dame, IN: Notre Dame University Press.

27 For an attempt to build a comprehensive theory of law and the work of lawyers, judges and legal theorists that makes extensive use of the concepts of interpretation and integrity, see Ronald Dworkin (1986) *Law's Empire*. Cambridge, MA: Belknap/Harvard University Press.

28 Edward Shils (1981) *Tradition*. Chicago: University of Chicago Press.

29 National Conference of Catholic Bishops (1986) *Economic Justice for All: Catholic Social Teaching and the U.S. Economy*. Washington, DC: United States Catholic Conference.

30 Ari L. Goldman (1986) 'Catholic bishops criticised on poor', *New York Times*, November 5, A20.

31. Jaroslav Pelikan (1984) *The Vindication of Tradition*, p. 81. New Haven, CT: Yale University Press.

9   Roman suicide

Miriam Griffin

Though advances in medicine have generated new problems demanding new techniques of moral reasoning, some problems of life and death were already subject to elaborate examination of this kind in the distant past. Thus a sophisticated type of argumentation was developed in classical antiquity to help with making moral decisions and moral assessments in the difficult area of suicide. Interest in such reasoning largely ceased, however, after AD 400 when, largely through the efforts of St Augustine, Christian doctrine became fixed in its total condemnation of suicide.

In the latter part of the nineteenth century, suicide started to become an important object of study to psychologists and sociologists, but their thinking has had little in common with the Greek and Roman approach, because both groups have regarded the act as something not fully understood or controlled by the victim. Lawyers, of course, had to worry about the precise determination of intention as long as suicide remained a criminal offence, but their concern with the avoidance of legal penalties led them to apply the formula 'when the balance of the mind was disturbed' so widely as to generate the belief that suicide could not be a rational act: in ancient thought, however, that situation was held to be the exception. In any case, the concern of the legal profession with such questions of motive has sharply diminished in England since 1961 when the law ceased to regard suicide or attempted suicide as an offence.

The current renewal of interest in practical ethics among English-speaking philosophers, however, makes the ancient approach relevant again, perhaps even useful. In particular, we may have something to learn from the study of the phenomenon that lies behind the tradition, still current, of 'the Roman cult of suicide', sometimes called simply 'Roman death'. This tradition has its roots in the detailed celebration in ancient literature of acts of suicide committed during the period when the Roman Republic gave way to a monarchical system and the first dynasties of Roman Emperors were on the throne.[1]

To catch the flavour of the phenomenon, let us consider three examples from the end of the first century BC and the first century AD, when the practice would appear to have been in its heyday.

First, the death of Titus Pomponius Atticus, a scholar and aesthete who was the favourite addressee of Cicero, Rome's greatest orator and prose writer. Though a late Republican figure, Atticus managed to survive almost to the end of the civil wars in which the Republic perished, finally putting an end to this life in 32 BC. His younger contemporary, friend and biographer, Cornelius Nepos, described what happened when Atticus, after suffering from a lengthy illness (apparently cancer of the bowel), decided to abstain from nourishment:

Feeling his suffering increase each day and attacks of fever beginning, he sent for his son-in-law Agrippa and with him Cornelius Balbus and Sextus Peducaeus. When he saw they had come, he said to them, leaning on his elbow, 'You have witnessed the unremitting care I have given to my health during this time, so that I need not remind you of it at length. These efforts, I hope, have satisfied you that I have neglected nothing that could cure me. It remains for me to consider myself. I wanted you to know that I have decided not to nourish my disease any longer. For during these last days, whatever food I have taken has just served to prolong my life, thereby increasing my suffering without hope of cure. Therefore I ask you first to approve my decision, then not to seek to hinder me by futile exhortation.' After this speech, delivered with such firmness of tone and expression that he seemed to be leaving one dwelling for another rather than leaving life, Agrippa begged him with tears and kisses not to hasten what nature would soon bring, and since he might even then survive the crisis, to preserve himself for himself and for those close to him, but Atticus met his pleas with stubborn silence (Nepos, *Atticus* 21–2).[2]

The second example is a suicide in a political context and belongs to the last terrible years of Nero's reign. In AD 65, some members of the upper classes formed a plot to kill the Emperor and replace him with a member of the old nobility. Seneca, the Stoic philosopher who had been an associate of Nero's for many years, first as tutor, then as adviser, was accused of complicity in the conspiracy because he had been on close terms with its leaders. He firmly denied the charge. We take up the account of the historian Tacitus, at the point when a praetorian officer has reported Seneca's denial to the Emperor, who asks:

whether Seneca was meditating suicide. Upon this the tribune asserted that he saw no sign of fear and perceived no sadness in Seneca's words or looks. He was ordered to go back and announce the death sentence . . . Seneca, quite unmoved, asked for tablets on which to inscribe his will. When the centurion refused his request, he turned to his friends, protesting that, as he was forbidden to reward them, he bequeathed to them the only thing he still possessed, yet the finest of all, – the pattern of his life . . . Then, he rebuked them for their tears, asking 'Where had their philosophy gone?' (*Ann.* 15.61)

The historian now recounts how Seneca and his wife severed their veins, after he had failed to dissuade her from joining him: 'Even at this last moment Seneca's eloquence did not fail him; he summoned his secretaries and dictated much to them which, as it has been published for all readers in his own words, I forbear to paraphrase.' (It is likely that these words were philosophical, perhaps about the immortality of the soul, as can be inferred from a suicide in the next year which imitated Seneca's in several respects.)[3]

Seneca, meantime, as the tedious process of death lingered on, begged his doctor to produce a poison which he had previously procured for himself, the same drug taken by those condemned by public sentence of the people of Athens (i.e. hemlock). It was brought to him and he drank, but in vain, for his limbs were cold and impervious to the poison ... At last he entered a bath of warm water from which he sprinkled the nearest slaves, saying 'I offer this liquid as a libation to Jupiter the Liberator'. He was then carried into a vapour-bath where he suffocated (*Ann.* 15.61–4).

Now certain common features of these deaths, different as they are, immediately strike us:

First there is the *theatricality* of these scenes, notably their length and the presence of a considerable audience. In Seneca's case, the suitability of the whole for literary treatment had already been exploited by the victim, who clearly knew that his last words would be published.

Then there is the *social character* of these deaths: friends are present, there is argument, comfort, attempted dissuasion.

Finally there is the *calmness* of the victim. His ostentatious lack of fear in the face of death is shown in the use of reasoned argument, the concern for others, and, in Seneca's case, the attention to the practical concern of his will.

These features already make a sharp contrast with what we still think of as the typical suicide of modern civilized countries, i.e. a solitary act expressive of despair and misery, with at most a brief suicide note to betoken social consciousness and to serve as a memento of the victim. Of course, there were suicides of that kind at Rome. For example, about thirty years before Seneca's death, a young man from one of the best families threw himself out of the window, because his mother had seduced him. Tacitus describes this as 'a sudden and undignified end'.[4] He despised the speed and the method alike, but he esteemed the sort of end that Seneca met. By contrast, the calm and deliberate suicide is still the exception, and the sociable type rare indeed: friends, if present, would feel obliged to hinder the attempt by force if necessary, and universal esteem afterwards cannot be assumed.

One explanation of the Roman attitude is suggested by a fourth feature of many Roman suicides, which we can see in Seneca's death, namely, their *philosophical overtones*. Seneca's allusion to the precepts of philosophy and his dictation of some for publication are obvious pointers. In fact the last discourse, the libation, and, above all, the allusion to hemlock, show us the influence of a definite philosophical model: Seneca's death was a re-enactment of the death of Socrates for which Plato, in his dialogue, the *Phaedo*, had provided the script.[5]

The philosophical overtones can be heard clearly in a briefer example which dates from the very end of the first century AD (97–8): the death of an elderly senator as lamented in a letter of his protégé Pliny. Corellius Rufus had suffered for many years from a painful condition of gout: 'As it grew steadily worse, he made up his mind to escape. Two days passed, then three, then four, but he refused all food.' At this point, Pliny was summoned by Corellius' wife and friends to dissuade him, but Corellius became more and more fixed in his resolve. Pliny comments:

Corellius, it is true, was led to make his decision by the supremacy of reason, which takes the place of necessity for the philosophers; but he had many reasons for living, a good conscience and reputation, and wide influence, besides a wife and sisters living, and a daughter and grandchild. In addition to so many close relatives, he had many true friends. But he suffered so long from such a painful illness that his *reasons* for dying outweighed everything that life could give him (Pliny, *Ep*. 1.12).

Here again we have the presence of an audience, the emphasis on giving reasons, the demonstration of calm and fearlessness, and the invocation of philosophy.

These last two examples show why the so-called 'cult of suicide' has commonly been explained as a consequence of the influence on the Romans of this period of the philosophy they had learned from the Greeks. Our first example, Atticus, was also a devotee of philosophy, that of Epicurus, but in committing suicide he was not following the mainstream of his school's teaching, as we shall see. That may explain why philosophy was not explicitly invoked by Atticus, though editing by his biographer, who disliked philosophy, cannot be ruled out.[6] Yet his calm and rational attitude was very much in keeping with Epicurean teaching, which stressed that death presented no terrors, being merely a return to nothingness.[7]

It is in fact Stoicism that is normally given the credit for making the practice of suicide acceptable, not only to members of that philosophical school but to society at large. Atticus was a true child of his time, for Epicureanism had a great vogue at the end of the Republic, but it was Stoicism that dominated the scene under the Empire. Its 'stiff upper lip' attitude accorded better with traditional Roman morality, which the first

Emperor, Augustus, was at pains to endorse. There was also another factor at work. While Stoicism and Epicureanism both emphasized the independence of the individual from external circumstances and were both good philosophies in adversity, Stoicism gave men dignity as well, and a feeling of moral superiority which compensated members of the upper orders for the political standing they had inevitably lost, now that a Princeps monopolized the power and the glory. According to the famous Stoic paradoxes, only the Stoic wise man was truly a ruler, truly an orator, truly rich, truly beautiful, truly free etc. What senator even in the old Republic could have aimed at a position as exalted as that? So Stoicism triumphed. For the upper classes living under the early Empire, Stoic philosophy can be thought of as fulfilling the role of Christian ethics in Western Europe even now. It provided a moral vocabulary and a framework even for those who were not believers, or knew its teachings only in a vulgarized form.[8]

Here is what the unsympathetic poet Martial has to say of the role of Stoicism in popularizing suicide:

In that you follow the maxims of great Thrasea and perfect Cato in such a spirit that you wish to live, instead of rushing with bared breast upon drawn sword, you act as I would have you act, Decianus. I have no use for the man who, by easy shedding of his blood, purchases fame; I value the man who can win praise, without death (I.8).

Cato and Thrasea were famous Stoic martyrs, and the charges of ostentation and glory-chasing made here were common ones levelled by the unsympathetic at Stoic adherents. Suicide was one occasion when these qualities would be particularly apparent. Indeed it is likely that the Roman jurist Ulpian had the Stoics particularly in mind when he identified a separate category of suicide as peculiar to philosophers. He lists the motives for suicide as: awareness of criminal guilt, disgust with life, intolerance of bad health – and finally, 'showing off, as with certain philosophers' (*Dig.* 28.3.6.7).

The idea of a 'Stoic cult of suicide' then has some claim to be considered, but great difficulties arise if the phrase is taken to imply that philosophy helped to change the attitude of the educated classes to suicide, from a predominantly condemnatory one to a more positive conception.[9] For, as we shall see,

(1) None of the philosophies popular in Rome at this time, including Stoicism, had anything more than a severely qualified approval of suicide to offer.

(2) It is clear that many kinds of suicide were already widely tolerated in Rome in the third and early second century BC, before the heyday of philosophical influence.

Before examining how the dominant schools viewed suicide (1), it would seem reasonable to consider briefly the word and its definition.

The word 'suicide' is derived from Latin but is not an actual Latin compound (*suus* not being used in compounds). In Latin, it would mean 'the killing of a pig'. The first use recorded in the *Oxford English Dictionary* dates from 1651, but in fact the word stands in the text of Sir Thomas Browne's *Religio Medici* (part I, ch. 44) as published by the author in 1643, and an instance has now been found in a French text of the twelfth century.[10] The Romans themselves resorted mostly to verbal phrases, the nearest to a technical term being *voluntaria mors*, 'a voluntary death'.

The most influential definition of suicide in recent times has been that offered by the French sociologist Emile Durkheim in his famous study of suicide, first published in 1897. Durkheim tried to define the phenomenon in sufficiently broad terms to embrace the variety of cases he wished to study: 'The term suicide', he wrote, 'is applied to any death which is the *direct* or *indirect* result of a *positive* or *negative* act accomplished by the victim himself, which he knows should produce this result.'[11] We are bound to feel that this definition covers such a large range of acts that, at the fringes, there are some that do not seem to be suicide at all. Thus the suicide by imperial command after sentence of death is a *positive* act whose *direct* result, as the victim knows, will be death, but we may feel that this is not suicide because the man has not chosen death as against life here, but merely one mode of death over another (execution). Again, Durkheim's definition covers heroic acts in war or acts of martyrdom, where death is the *indirect* result (through another agent) of an act performed by the victim which he knows will probably result in his death. But we may feel that this is not suicide, because the man's motive is not to end his life, but to adhere to some code of conduct and/or achieve some mission, even at the price of his life. The soldier who faces 'certain death', rushing into battle against overwhelming odds, or who throws himself on a grenade in order to save his companions, and yet survives, is rightly regarded as a hero, not as someone who has failed in his aim. Nor can his action normally be classified as a suicide attempt.

Durkheim was well aware of the broad scope of his definition, which arose principally from his deliberate rejection of the idea of *intention*. Indeed, he admitted that 'in common terms suicide is pre-eminently the desperate act of one who does not care to live', but he thought that any attempt to categorize acts by motivation was bound to founder on the fact that motive was difficult to ascertain even by a man observing himself.[12]

What interested Durkheim was *social causes*, that is social factors that made certain *groups* particularly liable to suicide, whether or not the individuals themselves were aware of these factors. But ancient thinkers were much more interested in moral decision and moral assessment than in social patterns. Hence the motive for suicide was usually specified by the ancient writers, even when they omitted other details, such as the method used. When they wrote about suicide they meant what the *Oxford English Dictionary* takes the word to mean in common use, i.e. 'the act of taking one's own life', a deliberate intentional act. Though the argument that the wish to kill oneself proves insanity does occur in a Roman rhetorical exercise, mental imbalance is rarely given as the cause of suicide, and then is usually seen as itself the product of a cause such as shame, which commonly motivates suicide, and is here the ultimate cause. Finally, the notion of intention was not complicated for the ancients, as it is for us, by the awareness of unconscious and subconscious motivation that we owe to psychology. Philosophers like J. Glover in *Causing Death and Saving Lives* (1977), may now prefer to speak of 'suicidal and near-suicidal acts' and to include among them, not only voluntary acceptance of a martyr's death (as Durkheim did), but volunteering for high-risk jobs where the '*risk* of death is welcomed or at least accepted with indifference' (pp. 170ff). On the other hand, the simple conception of a suicide attempt as a suicide that is stopped before death results, a conception that Durkheim shared with classical antiquity, now gives way to an awareness that some attempts are closer to real suicide in motive than others. One reason for refining our conceptions of motive here is an increasing concern with the moral problems of those in a position to prevent or not to prevent a suicidal act. They must consider not only, like the suicide himself, whether or not it is a rational decision which they can justifiably help to implement, but also what he really wants to do. But though many suicides in antiquity were carried out with assistance from others, notably slaves, those involved were spared that particular consideration.

It is time to turn to what the ancient philosophers had to say about suicide. The *locus classicus* at least in the period we are considering and later was the discussion between Socrates and Cebes in Plato's *Phaedo* (61 Cff.). There Socrates says that while any man devoted to philosophy must wish to die in order to free the soul from the flesh, he ought not to kill himself and desert the earthly service to which god has assigned him – unless the god sends some *necessity* (*anagke*) upon him. Such a necessity Socrates saw in the death sentence passed on him by the Athenians.

Now Socrates' drinking of the hemlock was actually a compulsory suicide, one of the borderline cases that fall under Durkheim's definition. Seneca, in fact, makes a contrast between Socrates' end and suicide, pointing out that Socrates could have ended his life in prison by abstaining from food but preferred to wait for the laws (*Ep.* 70.9). Earlier Cicero, who realized that Socrates was against suicide in the ordinary sense, had dismissed as typical Greek invention the story of Cleombrotus of Ambracia who leapt to his death simply because he had read the *Phaedo*.[13] As late as the fourth century the Emperor Julian, whose court orator Libanius compared the tent where he lay, surrounded by philosophers and dying of a battle-wound, to Socrates' prison (*Or.* 18.272), was able to comprehend the spirit of the *Phaedo*. In his farewell discourse, reported by the historian Ammianus (25.3), Julian thanked the gods for releasing his soul from his body, but then noted that it was cowardly and ignoble to solicit death when it was not right to die, or to decline it when the right moment came.

It is true that Plato in his later work, the *Laws* (9.873 C-D), was prepared to count as necessities justifying suicide, not merely the requirement of the laws (the case of Socrates), but painful and inevitable misfortune and irremediable and intolerable shame. And Aristotle allowed that to lay down one's life for friends or country could be noble (*NE* 9.1169a19ff.). But suicide as an escape from personal evils such as poverty, desire or pain he regarded as an example of cowardice (*NE* 3.1116a12); the suicide of the criminal as a sign of his justified self-contempt (*NE* 9.1166b10ff.) and suicide generally, except perhaps in the first (altruistic) case as an act of injustice against state (*NE* 5.1138a4ff.).[14]

Despite the predominantly negative view of Plato and his pupil, however, there is a kernel of truth in the story of Cleombrotus: that is the *impression* Plato's dialogue could make on the unwary reader, overwhelmed by its message of the immortality of the soul and its incarceration in the body.[15] This is one indication of the dilemma later faced by all the dogmatic Hellenistic schools of philosophy, namely that their insistence on the unimportance of external goods and of apparent evils like death, a doctrine designed to render life happy by making one independent of the blows of fortune, could in fact make life seem dreary and death attractive. Hence the Epicureans issued warnings against fleeing life because of hatred of life (D.L. 10.125–6; Lucr. 3.80), and the Stoics preached against the death wish (Sen., *Ep.* 24.24–5; Epictetus 1.9.12).

Naturally enough, it was the Cynics with their predominantly anti-social concept of virtue and their exaltation of individual freedom (D.L. 6.71) who placed the fewest restrictions on the right to commit suicide. They held that, since virtue is the only good, life is worth living for the wise man because he possesses it; there is nothing to tie the fool to life: their well-known dictum was 'Reason or the Rope' (Aelian, *VH* 10.11; D.L. 6.24). Yet, to put up with excessive pain due to illness, or old age or love might seem to place too high a value on life, so suicide was deemed acceptable in these cases (D.L. 6.18; 4.3; 6.86). It acquired a more positive function when used as a way of avoiding compulsion to act contrary to one's rational judgement of what it is right to do (Epictetus 4.1.30–1). Stoicism was to assimilate these last two ideas as part of a more sophisticated doctrine.[16]

The Epicureans, as we have said, were generally regarded as being against suicide. That emerges clearly from Seneca's story of the Epicurean philosopher Diodorus who was criticized for not following the doctrine of Epicurus when he took his own life (*Vita Beata* 19). The allegations of *dementia* and *temeritas* made by his critics echo the old idea much favoured by the Epicureans, that despair of life normally sprang from irrational fear of death, which it was their purpose to dispel (Xenophon, *Cyropaideia* 3.1.25; Seneca, *Ep.* 24.22–3). But the stumbling-block was pain, for they taught that the *summum bonum* of life was pleasure. Could one reject suicide as a release from pain? This consideration had induced one hedonistic philosopher, Hegesias, to preach the desirability of suicide, and to such effect that, according to Cicero (*Tusc.* 1.83), King Ptolemy of Cyrene had to ban his lectures fearing a drop in the population. But the Epicureans merely allowed that for those for whom the balance of pain over pleasure became intolerable, suicide was allowable (*Fin.* 1.49; 2.95). Even this solution was despised (Vat. frag. 9): the wise man ought, like Epicurus, to be able to maintain the balance of pleasure (mental of course) even in his last agonies (D.L. 10.22; Cicero, *Fin.* 2.96ff.).[17]

The Stoic theory of suicide was more elaborate.[18] For them, provided the *moment* and the *reason* were right, a man was justified in making a rational departure from life – the *eulogos exagoge*. They seem to have revered the view of Socrates, and their doctrine can be described as an internalization of Socrates' divine necessity so that it becomes a dictate of man's own reason, which tells him when life according to nature is no longer possible.[19] This modification of Platonism was made possible by the Stoic belief that the divinity of the world is immanent, consisting in its *logos* or reason, parts of which are present in man as his reason. In this way they licensed suicide in certain circumstances. Tradition held that Zeno, the founder of the Stoa, after a fall in which he fractured one of his digits, struck the ground with his hand and exclaimed, quoting from the *Niobe*, 'I come. Why do you call me?' He then held his breath and died (D.L. 7.28). Apparently he took the accident as a divine hint and committed suicide.

The Stoics devoted a lot of thought to what the acceptable reasons for committing suicide were. For them, all *kathekonta* (duties or appropriate acts) were acts for which a reasoned defence can be adduced (D.L. 7.107), but suicide belonged to a special class of duties, those imposed by exceptional circumstances (D.L. 7.109): for one's normal duty was to preserve one's life in accordance with the natural inborn instincts. Hence exceptionally strong reasons had to be found. One authority, Diogenes Laertius (7.130), states 'the wise man will make a rational exit from life, either on behalf of his country or for the sake of his friends, or if he suffers intolerable pain or mutilation or incurable disease'.

Another passage likens the proper reasons for leaving life to those for leaving a banquet (*SVF* 3.768):

(1) because the oracle tells one to kill oneself to save one's country; that is, in the simile, because one's services are suddenly required as in the case of the appearance of a friend after a long time;
(2) because tyrants are forcing us to do or say disgraceful things; that is, because of the arrival of rowdy revellers;
(3) protracted disease preventing the soul from using its tool, the body = spoilage of provisions at the banquet;
(4) poverty = scarcity of provisions at the banquet;
(5) madness = drunkenness at the banquet.

As these are all reasons for a rational departure from life, (5) must stand for perceived diminution of one's mental faculties through illness or age,[20] rather than a state of complete irrationality, which could be an explanation but not a justification.

All but the second obviously resemble the reasons given by Diogenes Laertius, which fall into two categories: the first category, corresponding to the first reason for leaving the banquet, is 'for the sake of his country and friends', which rests on the Stoic idea that a man has obligations to the community of rational beings to which he belongs. This sort of reason fits well with old Roman traditions of patriotism and loyalty which, we shall see, had even in early times rendered some types of suicide acceptable.

The second category 'pain, mutilation, incurable disease' corresponds to the third, fourth (and fifth) reasons for leaving the banquet and rests on the Stoic doctrine that, although virtue is the only good and vice the only evil, and everything else is indifferent, there are among the indifferents, positive ones (*proegmena*, things to be preferred) and negative ones (*apoproegmena*, things to be avoided). Death, pain, poverty are among the negative ones; life, pleasure, property, health among the positive ones (*SVF* 1.190). Life itself, like the others, has value only as material for virtuous action (*SVF* 1.399), so that the decision to retain life or not rests not, as for the Cynics, on the possession of virtue which is true happiness (*SVF* 3.758–60), but on the balance in life of the positive vs. the negative indifferents (*Fin.* 3.60): a sufficiently adverse balance means that virtuous action, which is the aim of life, will become severely impeded or impossible (*SVF* 3.763; 765–6). It was, of course, pain and mutilation that Zeno is supposed to have interpreted as a signal to die. He was then an old man and doubtless took the accident to show that his body was now so fragile as to impede a life of virtue (see Seneca, *Ep.* 30.2). Similar reasoning can be ascribed to the aged Cleanthes in the story that he refused to resume eating after two days of abstention which his doctors had recommended as treatment for severe inflammation of the gums (D.L. 7.176).

Now it will already be clear that much casuistry will have been necessary in deciding what a person's duty was in *any particular case*. How did one weigh up the balance of positive and negative indifferents? How could one best serve one's country and friends? Musonius Rufus (Hense frag. 29) held that dying could only be the duty of a man who was useful to many people, if his death could be useful to even more. And the two pointers to duty noted so far could offer apparently conflicting directives. Thus Seneca claims that it was Socrates' wish to go on serving his friends by philosophical discourse that led him to wait for the hemlock rather than commit suicide by abstinence in prison (*Ep.* 70.9), which would have spared him the prolonged agony of expectation and imprisonment.

There is still a third type of reason for suicide to be considered, one that corresponds to the second motive for leaving the banquet, i.e. 'because tyrants are forcing us to do or say disgraceful things'. One of the Stoic paradoxes pronounced that only the wise man is free. This freedom is not freedom in any material or political sense, but the freedom of the rational faculty from internal or external constraints in directing him to what is virtuous (D.L. 7.121). The wise man performs virtuous actions willingly, and wicked acts he cannot be forced to do (*SVF* 8.362–3; 544). To illustrate the Stoic paradox, philosophers had always given examples of men exercising freedom of speech before tyrants and defying death or torture rather than do disgraceful things (e.g. Epictetus 4.1).[21]

The paradox could obviously offer a justification for suicide in certain political circumstances, not of suicide *per se*, but of suicide as one way of accepting death as the price of preserving virtue. The paradox is really a justification of *martyrdom*, and Seneca and Epictetus clearly show no preference for suicide over martyrdom by execution in the right circumstances. Indeed at one point Seneca suggests that, even when faced with certain death, the sage may decide to wait for the executioner (*Ep.* 70.8). And Cato's suicide is regularly used simply to illustrate the wise man's contempt of death (Seneca, *Ep.* 24.6; 98.12).

None the less, as the Martial poem quoted earlier shows, there is much truth in the dictum of Arthur Darby Nock that suicide was in the first century AD 'the Stoic form of martyrdom *par excellence*'.[22] To understand why that should be so, however, we shall have to turn to history.

Before doing that, it is perhaps worth noting that once suicide is admitted into a system of rational morality, as some philosophers are now minded to do, the Stoic approach immediately appears viable again. Thus Jonathan Glover argues that simple acceptance of suicide as a matter for individual choice is as unsatisfactory as blanket disapproval; that questions about the quality of life and about obligations to family, friends and society must be weighed against one another; and that to allow this to be done properly, there should be discussion with others and an avoidance of acting too quickly.[23] Even the last category of Stoic suicide is catered for by Bernard Williams and Margaret Pabst Battin in the notion of 'fundamental ground-projects' which it is rational to pursue (or to avoid the frustration of) even at the cost of one's life.[24] These can include a certain conception of virtuous conduct, or honour, or even perfection in a skilled pursuit, often of a very individual kind comparable to the ideas of Panaetius (below, p. 121). Stoic ethics perhaps had an advantage over these views in being grounded on metaphysical principles about the nature of man. The Stoics were thus better able to distinguish individual 'ground-projects' from those appropriate to mankind in general, and to combine the idea of rational suicide with the notion that it must always be an exceptional course of action – a duty, but one only occasionally appropriate.

Just as suicide has been, and is, practised in all sorts of societies, from the most primitive to the most civilized, so there has probably never been a social code that sanctioned it absolutely *without conditions*. In primitive societies there are often deep-seated superstitions about *Biothanatol*, victims of violent or untimely death. It is a fear of the ghost, which it is thought will be vengeful or troubled and not rest in peace. Special modes of burial with denial of ordinary burial rites, originally an expression of this fear, are attested for Greece and possibly for early Rome. But whatever regulations of a religious kind once obtained in Rome, they seem to have lapsed by the historical period.[25]

Even apart from superstitious or religious considerations, it would be a rare community that would license its members to kill themselves regardless of circumstances, unless the community was bent on extinction: for in many cases, vital social obligations would be neglected through this act. But except for post-Augustine Christian and Muslim societies in which, at least in theory, suicide has been totally condemned, most societies have accepted certain types of suicide.

Of the types of suicide likely to be found socially acceptable, the most obvious would be suicides ordered by the state for the sake of preserving or protecting the society. Strabo records a primitive habit of this kind surviving into the fourth century BC on the island of Ceos in the Aegean

(10.5.6) where people over sixty were ordered to drink hemlock so that there would be enough food for the others. (It is interesting that Valerius Maximus (2.6.7–8) claims to have been the eye-witness of a voluntary suicide there by a woman of ninety in the reign of Augustus – which suggests that the tradition survived even when the law no longer obtained.) In some societies the death of widows and servants with their master has been mandatory, perhaps to make sure the ghost was satisfied and not tempted to trouble the living. The only form of suicide actually ordered by the state that we know of in Rome is the use of it as a form of death sentence: it is attested as early as 121 BC (Appian, *BC* 1.26).

Closest to suicides actually ordered by the state are those voluntarily undertaken to preserve it. We can regard in this light the ancient Roman practice of *devotio* whereby a general offered himself to the gods as a sacrifice in return for victory, and then plunged into battle to find death. Related to these are suicides undertaken to save others, such as the captain staying with his ship. Thus the Emperor Otho killed himself when victory was still possible, in order to stop civil war and the shedding of Roman blood (Tacitus, *Hist.* 2.47–50).

Next come suicides undertaken out of adherence to a social code of conduct, to avoid or make up for failure to meet social expectations: one can include here, for example, women preserving their chastity or atoning for its loss; generals anticipating defeat or killing themselves for shame; accused persons anticipating condemnation. The earliest suicides we hear of in Rome, besides practitioners of *devotio* and Lucretia who killed herself after being raped, are men forestalling legal condemnation[26] and military leaders avoiding the disgrace of defeat: credible historical examples go back to the second century.[27]

The use of a suicide order as a privileged form of capital punishment for upper class defendants already suggests that suicide was acceptable at least in educated circles by the late second century BC. (Those involved in government could regard the suicide of the accused as relieving them of the blood guilt (Dio 58.15).) By the first century AD there is stronger evidence for the general acceptability of suicide. In the reign of Tiberius, the law conceded to suicide in anticipation of condemnation the same privileges as were conceded to natural death, i.e. suicide prevented passage of sentence and thus confiscation of property and denial of burial (Tacitus, *Ann.* 6.29). One reason for the growing acceptance of suicide may have been the decline in superstitious belief in the afterlife (Cicero, *Tusc.* 1.48). For whereas Christianity was to offer, in its doctrine of the afterlife, some incentive to ending one's life, to which the traditional disapproval of the church served as counterweight, Roman religion offered little in the way of rewards after death. More imagination was lavished on Tartarus than on the Elysian Fields, so that the Elder Pliny (*NH* 7.55.190), who regarded suicide as the greatest gift given to man amid life's sufferings (*NH* 2.5.27), attacked the notion of an afterlife precisely for spoiling the greatest good offered by nature, namely death. Whereas for Christians the afterlife could encourage flight from life, for pagans it could only be a deterrent (Elder Seneca, *Controversiae* 8.4), especially as the traditional views on the afterlife enshrined the old distaste for suicide. The poet Virgil perhaps reflects the old and new attitudes when he places Cato in the Elysian Fields (*Aen.* 8.670), while relegating other suicides, with others cut off in their prime, to a gloomy place where they pine for the light (6.434ff.).

But despite the early evidence for tolerance, it has been claimed that as late as 46 BC, Caesar was assuming the vitality of the ancient repugnance for suicide when he chose to exhibit in his quadruple triumph pictures of the Pompeians who had killed themselves rather than surrender to him in Africa: they were shown in the very act.[28] But the historian Appian (*BC* 2.101) reports that grief was the response of the crowd, though fear restrained its expression. Moreover, in view of the facts collected above, it seems unlikely that Caesar could really have expected to turn the crowd against his enemies by stressing the mere fact of suicide: he seems to have felt it necessary to have them depicted in a gruesome way.[29] Finally, not only deaths by suicide seem to have been portrayed.[30] It is perhaps wrong to assume that Caesar was making a coolly calculated bid for popularity. The whole triumph over his fellow Romans was a tasteless performance, more plausibly motivated by resentment: for Caesar was peeved that his enemies had denied him the chance to demonstrate his famous clemency by pardoning them.[31] The pictures were a way of avoiding naming his fellow Romans, which would have been a gross breach of etiquette, but he was determined to have his victory over them after all!

Indeed these suicides fit into the pattern of those that had long been considered acceptable, namely, those to escape the shame of defeat and surrender.[32] This was true even of the most celebrated of them, that of M. Porcius Cato, Caesar's most consistent enemy who, after leading the resistance in Africa, declared that he was unwilling to be pardoned by Caesar because that would imply legal recognition of Caesar's position as tyrant through which he had acquired the power to save (Plut., *Cato Minor* 66).[33] That Cato died in the traditional situation of defeat was still remembered a century and a half later by the poet Martial who compared his death unfavourably with that of the Emperor Otho thus:

Although the goddess of civil strife still wavered and gentle Otho still had a chance to win, he cursed war that cost so much blood and with steady hand pierced deep his breast. Let Cato in life be greater even than Caesar: was he in death greater than Otho? (6.32)

Now Martial, as we have noted before, was hostile to Cato or rather to what Cato had become, namely, the solemnly revered and much-imitated model of heroic Stoic suicide.

When I suggested earlier that history alone could explain why suicide became in the early Empire the Stoic form of martyrdom *par excellence* (p. 116), I meant that it was the way in which the younger Cato chose to stage his end and the way in which others celebrated it thereafter that explain why political opponents of the Emperors, who were ordered to kill themselves or even were actually executed, came to be thought of, and probably thought of themselves, as following the great Stoic Cato in death. We have seen this assimilation in Martial's poem about 'great Thrasea and saintly Cato', though Thrasea actually opened his veins after capital sentence had been passed.[34] What helped blur these differences in the context of political martyrdom was, I suggest, Cato's self-identification with Socrates.

Every schoolboy, the poet Persius reminds us (3.45), had to recite the speech of the dying Cato, and one thing that was recounted by all of the rhetorical declaimers (Seneca, *Ep.* 24.6) and eulogists of Cato (including his Stoic biographer Thrasea Paetus) was his reading of the *Phaedo* on the night he died; in fact, according to Plutarch (*Cato Minor* 68.2; 70.1), he managed to read it through twice before midnight, before falling into a deep sleep. Towards dawn he awoke and stabbed himself. Cato thus identified himself with the dying Socrates and the significance of this was not lost.

The assimilation of the death of Cato to that of Socrates, so common in Roman authors, was made by the informed *not via* the concrete act of self-destruction – hemlock in the one case, the sword in the other – but *via martyrdom*: retaining the courage of one's convictions unto death (Seneca, *Cons. Helv.* 13.4–6; *Prov.* 3.4ff.; *Ep.* 13.14; 104.27ff.). For Socrates, as we saw, did not regard his death as suicide, and such men as Cicero and Seneca were well aware of that. In fact, Plutarch reports that Cato's nephew Brutus, who was, in philosophy, an adherent of Plato's school, at first regarded what Cato had done as impious, though he later changed his mind after Caesar's murder, and it must be against criticism of this sort that Cicero's curious remarks in the *Tusculan Disputations* (1.74), a work dedicated to Brutus, are directed.[35] There he notes that we should not leave life without an order from God and that Cato, like Socrates, was glad to be given a just cause by God.[36] If what we have said about Zeno and Cleanthes is right, Cicero was merely making explicit the comparison with Socrates *via* the divine hint that was implicit in their deaths.

Plutarch's account suggests that the Socrates of Plato's *Apology* and *Crito* was also in Cato's mind, Socrates the martyr, later celebrated by Cicero, in the same work, for seeking no advocate in his trial, for refusing to supplicate his jurors, for refusing to be rescued from prison and welcoming death instead (*Tusc.* 1.71 cf. *de Oratore* 1.231ff). That Cato's thoughts ran on these lines is shown by his animated defence on the fatal night of the Stoic paradox that only the wise man is free. It was this that led his friends to suspect his intention (67). Cato's death was, in fact, a rational exit from life according to the third type of reason the Stoa permitted.

We have returned by way of Cato to the question we raised earlier: is the fashionableness of suicide in the early Empire to be explained by the influence of philosophy? We have noted that there is evidence for widespread toleration of certain types of suicide at Rome before the period when philosophy became very influential; and that the most influential philosophy of the period demanded a high standard of ratiocination in determining if suicide in any particular case was the right thing to do.

We may further note that the Stoic philosopher Panaetius who had a great influence on Roman statesmen in the second century BC had made matters more difficult by developing the doctrine of *decorum*, according to which the inborn characteristics of an individual, his economic and social position and his chosen role in life might make an act appropriate for him, but inappropriate for another. An Olympic athlete would be right to accept death rather than physical mutilation through surgery, and a philosopher would be right to be martyred for his beard (Epictetus 1.2.25–9). Thus, according to Cicero, in a passage developing Panaetius' ideas, Cato was right to do what he did, but it would not have been the right course for his companions, for Cato's *constantia* was such that he could not, as the others could, appropriately adjust to the new political situation (*Off.* 1.112).[37]

None the less, Plutarch shows Cato himself having to dissuade some of his companions from imitating him then and there; many, like Cicero, felt compelled to justify themselves for not doing so.[38]

The most striking testimony to the power of Cato's example is found in another poem of Martial (1.78) in which he writes of a friend suffering from an incurable disease who did commit suicide under Domitian:

When wasting disease choked his guiltless throat and over his very face the black contagion spread, Festus, dry-eyed himself, gave heart to his weeping friends and

resolved to approach the Stygian lake. But he did not taint his righteous mouth
with hidden poison or with slow starvation torture his sad fate. His holy life he
closed with a Roman death and set free his soul by a nobler end. This death may
fame prize more than great Cato's doom; for Caesar was this man's friend!

That a man dying of disease should actually throw himself on his sword
and be celebrated as superior to Cato because of his politics is a
phenomenon that the mere popularity of Stoic philosophy in the early
Empire can hardly explain.[39] But it does allow one to claim that Stoicism,
not alone but via the powerful example of Cato, made suicide, not
tolerated or acceptable – for it was that already – but fashionable and
esteemed in the early Empire.

To understand why Cato's death had such a profound impact on
Roman upper class life – even outside Stoic circles – it is important to note
that the same political factors that made Stoicism so appealing also led to
an emphasis on dying nobly. Obituaries and death scenes of all kinds
abound in the literature of the early Empire, and we know of works that
dealt specifically with the deaths of famous men.[40] One plausible explanation of this emphasis lies in the restriction of the traditional opportunities
for acquiring glory that was imposed by the autocratic system of government. The Roman nobility found it more difficult to live up to the example
of their ancestors in acquiring military and civic fame, but they could still
die noble and memorable deaths. Suicide had a particular advantage in
this context, for it could be staged. One could make sure that one had an
audience and that one said memorable things. Only in opera is it usually
easy to achieve this with other forms of death.[41]

So philosophy, again via Cato, helped to provide *the etiquette and style*
for suicide. Not that we can guarantee that even the suicides described
actually measured up to the literary portrayal of them. Some literary
distortion may well have been customary, perhaps already in Plato. Thus
it has been persuasively argued that the gradual numbness that Socrates
experiences in the *Phaedo* bears little relation to the rather disgusting
symptoms of actual hemlock poisoning.[42] But life and literature here, as
elsewhere, probably exerted a reciprocal influence, literature improving on
life but also inspiring better performances.[43] Certainly, Roman jurists,
that hard-headed breed of men, thought, unlike Durkheim, that suicides
could easily be classified by motive (e.g. *Dig.* 3.2.11, 3; 48.21.3, 5–8) and,
though the motives they list include *taedium vitae* (weariness of life) which
no self-respecting philosopher would pass, their attitude suggests that
people commonly gave reasons to their friends and relations, just as they
do in the literary accounts.[44]

That it was the giving of reasons and the demonstration of fearlessness
in the face of death that was fashionable, and that philosophy played a

part in making them so is suggested, for example, by an Epicurean non-suicide scene, to which Seneca devotes an entire letter. The historian Aufidius Bassus was dying of old age, and his body was now so decrepit that, as Seneca says, he would have been justified (in Stoic terms) in deserting it (*Ep.* 30.2). Instead, he contemplated his inevitable but lingering end 'with a courage and countenance which you would regard as undue indifference in a man who so contemplated another's end'. Seneca goes on to say that those who meet death cheerfully and tranquilly can give us greater courage than those who seek death, for some have done that in a fit of rage. So Seneca went to visit Bassus frequently and listened to him discoursing at length on death in accord with the precepts of Epicurus. Thus an orthodox Epicurean could follow the fashion without committing suicide.

Pliny makes the points explicitly in a letter about the deliberations of his friend Titius Aristo (*Ep.* 1.22) on the question of suicide: 'Many people', he writes (para. 10), 'share his impulse and urge to forestall death, but the ability to examine and weigh the reasons for dying, and to accept or reject the idea of living or not, as reason urges, is the mark of a truly great mind'.

Some potential suicides, however, disliked the element of self-glorification in the long philosophical discourse and the imitation of Socrates and Cato. As a reaction, there developed the anti-philosophical tradition of death with panache. Here the fearlessness and rationality were shown by attention, not merely to ordinary matters like Seneca's will, but to the positively trivial. So Tacitus shows us Valerius Asiaticus checking the location of his funeral pyre before opening his veins, in order to ensure that the flames would not damage his trees (*Ann.* 11.3). But his triumph in this style is the death of Petronius, carried out on Nero's order and clearly regarded by victim and writer as the answer to the showing off of people like Seneca:

He severed his veins. Then, having them bound up again when it pleased him, he talked with his friends, but *not* about serious matters, with the aim of acquiring glory for his fortitude. And he listened to them reciting, *not* sermons about the immortality of the soul and the doctrines of philosophers, but light lyrics and frivolous poems. Some slaves received presents, – others beatings. He appeared at dinner and dozed, so that his death, even if ordered, should appear natural (*Ann.* 16.19).

Yet Socrates' last words in the *Phaedo*: 'We owe a cock to Aesculapius: pay it and do not neglect it' – even if Socrates is alluding to the philosophical view that life is a condition of sickness – show that the underplayed exit was not necessarily incompatible with philosophical discourse. In Seneca (*Tranq. An.* 14) we find a political martyr in the time of the Emperor Caligula juxtaposing the traditions of panache and philosophy. Julius Canus has a discussion on the immortality of the soul with his tame philosopher, but only after he has played draughts up to the moment of his summons to execution and then said to the soldier in charge: 'You will bear witness that I was one piece ahead.'[45]

So far we have made no effort to penetrate the vagueness of terms like fashionableness and cult. Do we mean that the actual number of suicides increased? We do not know; the ancient world did not keep such statistics. But we must recognize that the frequent use of suicide as a literary theme in the early Roman Empire may give us a false impression of an exceptionally high frequency of real suicides in this period. It has been plausibly argued that the extensive reporting of the history of this period by ancient writers and their wish to celebrate the courage and suffering of the Roman aristocracy in the transition from republic to monarchy accounts for this pattern.[46] It accords with this thesis that most of the suicides attested in the literary sources are those of members of the upper classes. We tend to hear of servile suicides only when they can be used to exhort or reproach their betters.[47] Only chance remarks suggest that less spectacular and heroic acts of suicide were commonplace at all social levels in this period, as when the Elder Pliny notes that the conditions which drive men to kill themselves are bladder-stones, stomach pains and headaches (in that order): he infers that these are the most painful of human ailments (*NH* 25.7.23).[48] It is clear that it would be rash to conclude that the suicide rate did increase, or that, if it did, it was more marked among the upper than the lower orders, though methods of suicide were to some extent socially differentiated.[49]

What does emerge from the celebration in literature of certain kinds of suicide is that the act, when performed in the right circumstances, was highly esteemed. What is esteemed will often be imitated, and we know that, in fact, stylish suicides often did find imitators. We have noted the zeal of Cato's companions, and Tacitus tells us that Otho's suicide was widely imitated in the military camps (*Hist.* 2.49). The wife of Thrasea Paetus wanted to emulate her mother Arria, who had killed herself in order to toughen her husband's resolve (Dio. 60.15.5–6; Pliny, *Ep.* 3.16).

We must then admit the possibility that the esteem attached to the rationally justified suicide and the publicity that literature gave to it may actually have made the act itself possible for many who, living at some other time, might not have resorted to it. One such man was the effete Neronian senator Caninius Rebilus, of whom Tacitus wrote (*Ann.* 13.30): 'He escaped the miseries of decrepit old age by opening his veins. Because of his notorious effeminacy, no one had thought he had the courage to kill himself.'

NOTES

This chapter is a revised version of M. T. Griffin (1986) 'Philosophy, Cato, and Roman Suicide'. *Greece and Rome* 33: 64–77; 192–202.

1 Y. Grisé (1982) *Le suicide dans la Rome antique* (Montreal-Paris) the first collection of evidence devoted exclusively to Rome. The most complete collection of material on Greek and Roman suicide remains R. Hirzel (1908) 'Der Selbstmord', *Archiv für Religionswissenschaft* 11: 75–104, 243–84, 417–76. The recent *From Autothanasia to Suicide* (London) by A. J. L. Van Hoof (1990) analyzes cases of suicide in Greek and Roman sources as a key to popular moral attitudes with less emphasis on philosophical views.

2 This obituary, part of the epilogue (19–22) which was added in a second edition of the Life, was composed before the conferment on Octavian of the title 'Augustus' in 27 BC, thus within five years of Atticus' death.

3 Thrasea Paetus' death: Tacitus, *Ann.* 16.34–5. For this view of Seneca's last words, see M. T. Griffin (1976) *Seneca* (Oxford) pp. 370–1.

4 *Ann.* 6.49. This mode of death was regarded as dishonourable and was often associated with shame in a sexual context (A. J. L. van Hooff (1990) *From Autothanasia to Suicide* (London) pp. 74–5).

5 Tacitus underlines the conscious imitation by noting that Seneca took hemlock, of which he had secured a supply in advance (*Ann.* 15.64.3), and by describing it as 'the poison used to put to death those condemned in the public court at Athens'.

6 Atticus' Epicureanism: Cicero, *ad Att.* 4.6.1; *Leg.* 1.21; 54; 3.1; *Fin.* 5.3. Nepos speaks of Atticus' knowledge of the teachings of the leading philosophers which he used as a guide for life, not for ostentation (17.3), but does not specify Epicureanism any more than he does for L. Saufeius and Lucretius, known Epicureans (12.3–4). Nepos had no use for philosophy (Cicero, *ad Att.* 16.5.5), because of the hypocrisy of its adherents (Lact., *Inst.* 3.15.10), and perhaps disapproved of Epicureanism in particular. It is all the more striking that, as C. Bailey pointed out (*JRS* 41 [1951], 164), there are incidents recorded in language suggestive of Epicureanism: *tranquillitas* at 6.5; *quies* at 7.3; and at 6.1 (see also 10.5–6), in explaining Atticus' failure to enter public life, Nepos uses nautical imagery which, though in no way exclusive to the sect (see, e.g. Cicero, *Off.* 3.2), is very reminiscent of Lucretius 2.1–2 and of Cicero's version of the Epicurean doctrine of abstention in *Rep.* 1.1.4; 9.

7 Nepos does not, however, stress the Epicurean overtones. Instead he speaks of Atticus' *constantia*, a Stoic quality, while the phrase he uses to describe the impression made on Atticus' companions, 'that he seemed to be leaving one dwelling for another, rather than leaving life', if it has any philosophical significance, is suggestive, not of Epicureanism, but, as Harrison (1986) points out in *Classical Quarterly* 36: 505, of Plato's *Apology* and *Phaedo*, especially as rendered by Cicero, *Rep.* 6.15: 'nor must we depart from the life of men except at the command of the one who gave us our soul' and 6.29: 'a spirit so trained will have a swifter flight to this, its proper abode and permanent home', see also *Hortensius* frag. 115 Grilli. Nepos uses the image of moving house, to convey the idea of insouciance as in Horace, *Odes* 3.5.55–56, a passage

probably indebted to Cicero, *Fin.* 2.65 and hence having some Epicurean resonance.

8 On the flexibility of Stoicism and its importance in providing terminology and arguments, rather than definite directives, especially in political matters, see *Seneca,* p. 366, 204–5. B. D. Shaw, 'The Divine Economy: Stoicism as Ideology', *Latomus* 44 (1985) makes similar points on pp. 48ff.

9 The phrase 'Stoic cult of suicide' is found in A. D. Nock (1933) *Conversion* (Oxford) p. 197. H. R. Fedden (1938) *Suicide, a Social and Historical Study* (London) p. 85 speaking of Stoicism and Epicureanism, wrote 'Physical courage and the state of society needed only the stimulus of philosophy to elevate suicide to the place and popularity which it enjoyed in the time of Seneca.'

10 'Yet herein are they (viz. the Stoics) in extreams that can allow a man to be his own assassine and so highly extol the end and suicide of Cato.' D. Daube (1972) in his influential paper 'The linguistics of suicide', *Philosophy and Public Affairs* 1: 387ff. not only credits the first use of the word to W. Charleton (1659) in *The Ephesian Matron* but suggests it was invented to avoid expressing condemnation. But Charleton probably copied the word from Browne who liked adding technical terms to the language (such as 'electricity' and 'computer') and who consistently, in this passage and elsewhere, disapproved of suicide. I owe this information to Dr. Robin Robbins, who also points out that Charleton makes clear his disapproval of the soldier's soliloquy in which the word is used and employs 'self-slaughter' in the same context. For the twelfth century example, see A. J. L. van Hooff (1990) *From Autothanasia to Suicide* (London) p. 271, n. 4.

11 'On appelle suicide tout cas de mort qui résulte directement ou indirectement d'un acte positif ou negatif, accompli par la victime elle-même et qu'elle savait devoir produire ce résultat.'

12 The ancient writers themselves show that the difficulty Durkheim pointed to is a real one and that the criterion of motive will not enable suicide to be distinguished from martyrdom unambiguously. Thus Clement of Alexandria, one of the earliest Christian writers, complains that those Christians who parade their beliefs in such a way as to provoke Roman governors to put them to death are suicides, not, as they claim, martyrs (*Stromata* 4.4: 17.1) – that is, they really desire to die, not just to remain faithful to their beliefs. On the other hand, Roman writers who make no distinction between obvious suicides like Cato and upholders of freedom who die by compulsory suicide or even execution clearly regard the former more as martyrs than as suicides.

13 Cicero found the story in an epigram of the Greek poet Callimachus (A. S. F. Gow and D. L. Page (1965) *The Greek Anthology: Hellenistic Epigrams* (Cambridge), Callimachus no. 53 (= Pfeiffer 23). See also Cicero. *Scaur.* 4–5: *Tusc.* 1.84.

14 In this obscure passage, Aristotle does not seem to be placing in the category of injuries to the state, only suicides committed in anger (as Y. Grisé (1982) *Le suicide dans la Rome antique* (Montreal-Paris) p. 173 thinks), but using them as an example of how a man might come to kill himself voluntarily (see Seneca, *Ep.* 30.12).

15 Josephus was able to use Plato's arguments, in his own speech, against suicide (*BJ* 3.371ff.) but also, in the mouth of Eleazar, in favour of it (*BJ* 7.343ff.).

16 For a discussion of Cynic views of suicide, see J. M. Rist (1969) *Stoic Philosophy* (Cambridge) pp. 237–8.

17 Y. Grisé (1982) *Le suicide dans la Rome antique* (Montreal-Paris) p. 177 interprets Epicurus' death, as described by Hermarchus (D.L. 10.15), as suicide. But it is better to assume that the warm bath and wine were used to ease a natural end, in view of the general reputation of the School and the discussion in *Fin.* 2.95–8 where Cicero opposes to the recommendation of suicide an Epicurean formula and then quotes Epicurus' dying claim that his pains were counterbalanced by his joy, comparing Epicurus to Epaminondas and Leonidas. In the same vein is Epicurus' dictum that the wise man will not withdraw from life even when he has become blind (D.L. 10.229).

18 The best discussions are by A. Bonhoeffer (1894) *Die Ethik des Stoikers Epictet* (Stuttgart) pp. 29–39; E. Benz (1929) *Das Todesproblem in der Stoischen Philosophie* (Tübinger Beiträge zur Altertumswissenschaft 68), pp. 48ff.; J. M. Rist (1969) *Stoic Philosophy* (Cambridge) pp. 233ff. who rightly criticizes Benz' notion that suicide was seen by the early Stoics as a problem of free will. In M. T. Griffin (1976) *Seneca* (Oxford) pp. 372ff., I have tried to show that Seneca's view of suicide was much more in accord with orthodox Stoic doctrine than Rist then allowed. (See p. 517 of Postscript to the 1992 paperback edition of *Seneca*.)

19 I follow J. M. Rist (1969) *Stoic Philosophy* (Cambridge) pp. 242–5 in thinking that Zeno was conscious of a parallel with the death of Socrates, though Plato's *Phaedo* is not attested in theoretical discussions of suicide before the time of Cicero. For that reason, E. Benz (1929) *Das Todesproblem in der Stoischen Philosophie* (Tübinger Beiträge zur Altertumswissenschaft) pp. 71ff. suggested that the notion of a divine call came in with Panaetius and Posiodonius who were sympathetic to Plato's teachings. But tradition held that Zeno had a boyhood interest in reading about Socrates (D.L. 7.31), while the Callimachus epigram (above, n. 13) shows that the connection of the *Phaedo* and suicide was made earlier.

20 As in Seneca, *Ep.* 58.36; see also Marcus Aurelius, *Med.* 3.1.1.

21 For the difficulties involved in reconciling this doctrine with the Stoic view that the intention behind an action, not its result, is what matters, see M. T. Griffin (1976) *Seneca* (Oxford) pp. 380–1.

22 A. D. Nock (1933) *Conversion* (Oxford) p. 197.

23 J. Glover (1977) *Causing Death and Saving Lives* p. 197.

24 M. Pabst Battin (1982) *Ethical Issues in Suicide* (New Jersey) pp. 146ff. discussing B. Williams (1976) 'Persons, Character and Morality', in A. Rorty (ed.) *The Identities of Persons* (California) pp. 197ff.

25 Greece: Arist., *NE* 5.1138a13; Aeschines, *Ctes.* 244; Rome: Servius on *Aen.* 12.603; Pliny, *NH* 36.24, 107 though the sanction may have been limited to suicide by hanging: see Y. Grisé (1982) *Le suicide dans la Rome antique* (Montreal-Paris) pp. 127–56. On the Roman contempt for hanging as a method, see A. J. L. van Hooff (1990) *From Autothanasia to Suicide* (London) pp. 66ff.

26 E.g. Appius Claudius the decemvir: Livy 3.58.6; C. Papirius Carbo in 119 BC: Cicero, *Brutus* 103.

27 E.g. P. Crassus Mucianus in 131 BC (V. Max. 3.2.12); M. Aemilius Scaurus in 102 BC (V. Max. 5.8.4), cf. Cicero, *Sest.* 48.

28 J. Bayet (1951) 'Le suicide mutuel dans la mentalité des romains', *L'Année Sociologique*, 44, accepted by P. Jal (1963) *La guerre civile à Rome* (Paris) p. 173 and R. MacMullen (1967) *Enemies of the Roman Order* (Cambridge, MA) p. 5.

29 Cicero, when he first heard of the deaths of the Republicans in Africa in July of 46 (before the celebration of the triumphs in the autumn), wrote 'the others, Pompey, your friend Lentulus, Scipio, Afranius, came to miserable ends. But Cato's, you say, was splendid' (*Fam.* 9.18.2). The others mentioned had been murdered but Metellus Scipio committed suicide by stabbing himself and falling overboard when his ship was about to be captured, and, in later writers (Seneca, *Ep.* 24.9–10; Quintilian 5.11.10), his death is celebrated as comparable to Cato's. It is possible that Cicero did not yet know the circumstances of his death, on which our evidence is discrepant. He may have thought he had been killed (as implied in *B. Afr.* 96.2) or that his suicide had been accomplished by drowning (as in Livy, *Per.* 114), a means not esteemed by the Roman upper classes (Y. Grisé (1982) *Le suicide dans la Rome antique* (Montreal-Paris) p. 113). Alternatively, he may already have decided that suicide in these circumstances was only appropriate to Cato because of his character, as he says in *Off.* 1.112, where, however, the contrast is drawn only with those who surrendered.

30 As is suggested by the fact that Appian, *BC* 2.101 comments on the omission of Pompey's death from this exhibition. This omission is not a reason for seeing in Caesar's action a bid for popular favour rather than a display of vindictiveness, for, though Appian may be right to emphasize Pompey's popularity in this context, it was more relevant that he had been killed by Egyptians (not by Caesar) – their punishment was displayed. The defeat of the allied city of Massilia was also put on show (Cicero, *Phil.* 8.6.18).

31 Amply attested in the case of Cato: Appian, *BC* 2.99; Plut., *Cato Minor* 72.2; *Caesar* 54; Dio 43.12.1.

32 In view of the long tradition, not only Roman but foreign, of suicide in the face of defeat that Y. Grisé (1982) *Le suicide dans la Rome antique* (Montreal-Paris) demonstrates, it seems an odd suggestion that Caesar expected the crowd to view these suicides as a desertion of military duty (pp. 164, 270).

33 See also Elder Seneca, *Con.* 10.3.5; *Suas.* 6.2; Dio 43.10.3 whose interpretation is even less philosophical.

34 The parallels between Cato's death and that of his biographer Thrasea Paetus, both in reality and in the literary representations, and their relation to Socrates' death and its celebration in the *Phaedo* are well brought out by J. Geiger (1979) 'Munatius Rufus and Thrasea Paetus on Cato the Younger', *Athenaeum*, 57: 61–5.

35 Plut., *Brutus* 40.4ff. (*me hosion* echoes *Phaedo* 62A). Brutus was an adherent of the Old Academy, a Platonist in the new dogmatic style introduced by Antiochus of Ascalon (Cicero, *Brutus* 149, 332; *Fin.* 5.8). Florus (2.17.15) curiously explains the assistance of others at the deaths of Brutus and Cassius as a means of remaining true to 'their philosophical creed' (Cassius was, in fact,

an Epicurean) in that 'for the destruction of their brave and pious lives, they used their own judgement, but the hands of others to execute the crime'.

36 When Cicero first heard of Cato's death, he described it as 'necessary' (*Fam.* 9.18.2), but this is probably not an allusion to Socrates' *anagke* but shows that Cicero either did not know or did not credit Caesar's wish to pardon Cato (above, n. 31). By the time he wrote *De Officiis*, after Caesar's murder, he seems to have believed it (as 1.112 implies) and to have found another justification for his own failure to commit suicide like Cato (see below, n. 38).

37 For the importance of the doctrine of *personae* in this context, see *Seneca*, pp. 381–2. Cato seems to have made the distinction himself: Appian, *BC* 1.98; Dio 43.10.5; Plut., *Cato Minor* 64.3–5; 65.4–5; 69 (in speaking to his philosophers).

38 Plut., *Cato Minor* 65.4; 66.4; Cicero, *Fam.* 9.18.2 (see above, n. 36); 7.3.4; 4.13.12.

39 The sword is here preferred as a 'Roman death', though poison and starvation were not generally despised by the Roman upper class, as the examples of Atticus, Corellius Rufus and Seneca show. Probably it was felt to be the appropriate method for soldiers and commanders (as Cato was at the time): note the suicide of a Roman soldier by the sword celebrated as a victory over disease in Greek epigrams of the first century AD (*AP* 7.233 = Gow-Page (1968) *Garland of Philip* (Cambridge) Apollonides 20; *AP* 7.234 = Gow-Page, (1968), Philip 31; also relevant is *AP* 9.354 = Page, Leonidas of Alexandria 31). This might support the identification of Martial's Festus with C. Calpetanus Rantius Quirinalis Valerius Festus who had a distinguished military career.

40 Pliny, *Ep.* 5.5; 8.12.4; note his own efforts in this vein: 3.16; 6.16; 7.19.

41 The death of Cato in April of 46 BC was already described by Cicero in his *laudatio* (Elder Seneca, *Suas.* 6.4) which he started to write in May or June (*Att.* 12.4), and in extended form, for it seems to have included Cato's attempt to dissuade his son and Statillius from imitating him (Priscian, *GLK* II 510.19). It must also have been treated in the other eulogies and attacks on Cato including one by the Epicurean Fabius Gallus (*Fam.* 7.24.3). All of this literary activity may be the inspiration behind Nepos' extended treatment of Atticus' death which already exhibits some of the classic features of the later literary tableaux.

42 C. Gill (1973) 'The Death of Socrates', *Classical Quarterly* 23: 25ff.

43 Cato's irascible conduct, contrary to Stoic teaching, which surfaces at times in Plutarch's account (*Cato Minor* 67.2; 68.3–5) and was emphasized by E. Benz (1929) *Das Todesproblem in der Stoischen Philosophie* (Tübinger Beiträge zur Altertumswissenschaft) p. 118, helps to guarantee the truth of the account for which Plutarch's immediate source was Thrasea Paetus. His ultimate sources could include eye-witness accounts.

44 The jurists for the period from Trajan on were concerned, for financial reasons, to exclude from the legal privileges that death before condemnation could secure, suicides carried out in consciousness of guilt and expectation of condemnation. Therefore they were often content to lump respectable reasons such as illness, poverty, shame under the heading *taedium vitae*. This usage is akin to that of Latin writers generally (e.g. Pliny, *NH* 2.63.156) and is distinct from the philosophers' use of the phrase to condemn an irrational distaste of life (Seneca, *Ep.* 24.22; 78.25). This is discussed by Y. Grisé (1982) *Le suicide dans la Rome antique* (Montreal-Paris) pp. 72–3; 259.

45 The promise to tell his friends what he discovered about the nature of the soul through dying was carried out in a further elaboration of the story in Plutarch, *Mor.* frag. 211 S.

46 A. J. L. van Hooff (1990) *From Autothanasia to Suicide* (London) pp. 11–14. Y. Grisé (1982) *Le suicide dans la Rome antique* (Montreal-Paris) pp. 53–7, however, believes there was an increase in the suicide rate between *c.* 100 BC to AD 100, but only among the members of the upper classes whose lives were most affected by the political upheavals of the period.

47 Seneca uses examples of servile suicide to illustrate contempt for death even among the lowly (*Ep.* 70.19ff.; see also 24.11): the suicide of an ex-slave of Augustus' daughter Julia (Suetonius, *Aug.* 75.2) and that of the ex-slave Epicharis (Tac., *Ann.* 15.57) are used to show up ignoble conduct by their social superiors. See now the collection of evidence on lower class suicide in A. J. L. van Hooff (1990) *From Autothanasia to Suicide* (London) pp. 16–20; 166.

48 Inscriptions, papyri and technical writings (to which the Elder Pliny's encyclopedia is akin) can be more revealing in this respect. The possibility of suicide, always a problem for insurance schemes, was worth mentioning in the regulations for the burial club at Lanuvium in AD 136 (*ILS* 7212, II. 3–4): members of such clubs were men of modest means, slave and free.

49 Hanging, drowning and jumping off heights were normally eschewed by the upper classes, apparently because they were disfiguring (A. J. L. van Hooff (1990) *From Autothanasia to Suicide* (London) pp. 77–8).

10   Women and children first

Grant R. Gillett

The cry 'Women and children first!' is hallowed in both maritime history and moral tradition. There are many incidents similar to the Zeebrugge disaster in which folk have died attempting to save young children and those weaker than themselves. But the deep-rooted intuition this cry expresses is suspect in moral formulations where we attempt to justify assigning moral properties to various actions, states of affairs and beings of this or that kind. It soon emerges that the most obvious justifications available to us fail to give any especial weight to the claims of infants and children. This should prompt us to ask whether it is our moral intuitions or our moral formulations that need revision.

I will examine the basis for our special concern for the young and helpless and argue that it is basic to our nature as ethical beings. This suggests that many of our moral justifications fail to capture the essence of moral thought. I will argue that our moral reasoning about beings of various kinds is based on something close to 'reactive attitudes'[1] rather than the objective properties of those subjects (although mental ascriptions play a pivotal role in the story).

(1) We intuitively believe that the ethical importance of a human being is greater than that of an animal, plant or computer. To justify this judgement as being more than just an irrational prejudice in favour of human beings, we usually invoke facts about the wishes and desires of the individuals concerned, their conscious appreciation of life and/or their preferences about what should happen to them. But, on any set of criteria of this type, it is plain that neonates and certain mentally defective children turn out to be less-well-qualified candidates for ethical consideration than animals such as chimpanzees, gorillas, perhaps dolphins and maybe even pigs. It is however abhorrent to us, and, I should think, particularly disturbing for a paediatrician, to be told not to worry about the death of an infant or neonate because it is of no more consequence than that of a family pet. A moral theory based on mental properties suggests just this sort of parity because the intellectual functions, desires and interests of an infant are similar to those of a higher animal. What is

more, someone firmly convinced by such a view might hold that it was more morally defensible to do medical research on selected infants and neonates than on laboratory animals which are 'superior' to them in cognitive function. But, however well argued this view may seem to be, most people feel that it cannot be right. It remains to show why. In doing so we should show what is is about moral thought that explains our special regard for infants and that it is consistent with the fact that moral reasoning is *reasoning*.

(2) Why *do* we bother with neonates, even premature ones and treat it as a tragedy if we see one of these tiny human organisms die? We cannot understand the badness of death in terms of the individual's preferences and hopes for the future because an infant does not have such attitudes. In fact he does not have much to lose in terms of his actual experience and thought-life. On the other hand we could say that he has a great deal to lose because of his potential to become a fully morally valued human being. This is not just the argument that he has, potentially, a number of years ahead of him to enjoy. Indeed this (consequentialist) view depends on children being given the status and entitlements (to have their future prospects respected and so forth) of full-blown members of the moral community. That, however, is just what is in dispute. The argument from potential has its problems in that it is hard to say just when one should begin to count that potential as sufficient to outweigh other moral considerations.[2] If the potential to be a human being does confer special moral status on an individual then we will need to regard that potential as more than just a prediction that a being of a certain type (which lacks certain morally relevant properties) will turn into a being of another type. The view of potential we need is one which regards potential as an inherent property of a being of a certain type such that we should look at that individual as a total being whose nature is revealed over time and development rather than a being whose attributes are all present at any single point in time. If we took that view then the evident moral value of adult human beings would confer value on the child as well. However it would not account for our special regard for children.

We need to meet the challenge that this is just an emotive response toward the young of our own species and therefore uncomfortably close to racism or bigotry of other kinds.[3] There is no doubt that we do regard it as morally commendable rather than just foolish to prefer infants and their weal when a group of human beings is threatened by a common danger and we do regard human infants as being of greater moral value than those of other species.

In fact, our problem has a further twist. A significant amount of paediatric time and effort goes into saving and nurturing children who are weak and sickly *either* through some identifiable genetic problem such as oesophageal atresia, PKU, Down's syndrome, spina bifida, or oxalosis *or* for other less well-defined reasons. But ought we to do this kind of thing? If we argued that an austerely rational ethics should value above all the survival of humankind as a successful species, then the survival, perhaps to reproductive age, of defective or weak children can only influence the gene-pool in undesirable ways. Therefore, although this is shocking at first sight, nothing should be done to promote the survival of such defective individuals.

Similarly, any approach which predicated moral value on that which promotes the greatest happiness for the greatest number, could recommend such a stance. The survival of defective children involves the use of precious resources on individuals who are never going to lead full and healthy lives and it may positively discourage the affected families from having other children who (a) would not use those resources and (b) would lead more fulfilled lives. What is more, reproduction by such children will only lead to more lives as defective as their own and so not only multiply the negative values present in the situation but do it at great medical and social cost.

Some 'Kantian' positions yield a similar conclusion.[4] Children are not fully rational and participating members of the kingdom of ends and therefore do not deserve the same consideration as other human beings. They therefore have moral value only because other human beings, who do qualify for full moral consideration, have certain attachments to them. This implies that infants have no intrinsic moral worth over and above the attitudes of those other (adult) beings who 'own' them (in the sense of being the source of their moral status). Thus we have indirect moral duties to children but no direct duties to the children themselves. But our attitudes seem to concern the infant *per se* and not just the feelings of other moral agents because we regard a parent's wishes as infinitely more important than those of the owner of a pet, to the point where the former are expected to be extreme and uncompromising on matters touching their children but the latter are regarded as eccentric if they reach the same intensity.

These arguments run directly against the powerful but, so far, unsupported intuition that a child is valuable in itself and that to respond morally to an afflicted infant is commendable. Our intuition seems to go even further in that many would regard it as moral destitution of a particularly blatant kind to ignore the well-being of an infant. But does this stress on our sentiments imply a subjectivist account of moral reasoning? The moral theorist, in objecting to this can concede that it is understandable that we do feel this way toward children – it is probably instinctive and biologically based – but argue that as moral thinkers we cannot be pawns of instinct and must define what we *should* do in moral matters. We should choose our 'oughts' on rational or at least reasoned grounds such that principles, not feelings, form the foundation of sound ethics.

I will examine the rational foundation for moral reasoning and argue that *moral sense* is fundamental to the content of moral judgement in general. I will argue that moral facts are not determinable independently of the moral judgements of competent moral agents. This implies that we cannot afford to ignore the moral intuitions of those agents except where they are clearly disordered. We are forced to an alternative view of what is reasoned and informed in ethics, one that coheres well with the fundamental impulse of medicine. When applied to the special concern we have for children and the tragedy of infant death this account of moral reasoning explains why situations do and should catch us at the point where we are most human.

(3) First we need to examine the (Humean) divide between the rational and the intuitive aspects of our thought. Thoughts and arguments rest on concepts – some simple, like the concept 'red', and some rather complex, like 'Paris'. The basis of concept use is the ability to judge whether a concept is applicable in a certain situation and to inform and guide one's activity in the light of that ability.[5] In our moral thinking we use all sorts of concepts like 'kind', 'cruel', 'good', 'right' etc. To be competent in using such concepts is fundamental to moral understanding and reasoning. But now a curious fact emerges. When we make judgements about whether things are red, square or moving (all of which are quite objective) there is only a certain amount that reason can do (as Kant astutely noted). If a potential user of such concepts cannot 'latch on' to the rule we apply after we have shown him a number of instances then we are stuck. We cannot make up for his deficiency by using arguments and must fall back on something like 'But can't you *see* that they are all the same in a certain way?' Kant refers to this as 'mother wit', defects of which cannot be redressed by reason even though an individual's conceptual competence (and thus his reasoning) depend on it. If he cannot see what is meant by calling something 'square' then he cannot begin to reason about the properties of squares on the basis of his own experience. His defect lies in the fact that he cannot (to use a well-worn phrase) 'go on in the same way' or catch on to the rule for judgement that we all find so natural to apply in these situations.[6] (This naturalness is, clearly, an important factor in grasping a concept and may explain why Wittgenstein says he is 'making remarks on the natural history of mankind'.)[7]

We can illustrate this by imagining a case where you and another person have a chance to observe a family interaction and you see an infant drop an ashtray with which it is playing. The father gets out of his chair and starts hitting the child, shaking it and throwing it around. The infant is crying but the man goes on until he kicks the child across the room. You say to your companion 'How could anyone be so cruel?' He says 'What do you mean?' You attempt to explain but although he agrees about what happened he does not understand why it is cruel. One is surely entitled to conclude, *ceteris paribus*, that this person lacks something basic to a normal human understanding of the situation. In the end one might just have to fall back on the appeal 'But can't you see?' as in the case of a colour, a shape, or the detection of movement.

There are two possibilities which can account for your companion's failure of moral judgement and they clarify what is at stake in moral thought. He could say 'That is not cruelty because . . .' (detailing some set of reasons supporting an alternative interpretation), or 'I do not see what concerns you'. The first involves facts which mitigate or change the nature of the case. In the case described it would seem that no such facts could suffice – whatever else is going on, the actions still come out as being morally unacceptable. Therefore it seems that the observer just does not respond in the way required to grasp the concept 'cruel'. He appears to lack a basic recognitional ability necessary for the detection of those features of the situation that ground the judgement.[8]

So, our first move against a 'narrowly rational' view of moral justification is to claim that the abilities we habitually exercise in thought all rest on our natural sensitivities, reactions and responses to what goes on around us. This, as some may have realised, is a point made not only by David Hume but also by Wittgenstein and Strawson.

(4) If natural sensitivities are basic to both general and moral thought, then what sort of reactions, and propensities underpin moral judgement?

As a first attempt to identify the grounds of our moral judgements, we might claim that it is intellect or cognitive capacity that matters in determining which beings have ethical value. This distinguishes humans from slugs and beetles but has problems when we get to computers whose purely 'intellectual' functions may be superior to ours in some respects. And there is no obvious reason why the ability to crunch large amounts of data should be morally significant. (Notice that we are in some doubt as to whether we should say that such a machine is thinking or merely 'information processing'.)

We can clarify things further by imagining a robot which achieved, by whatever means, the ends that cold and callous calculations dictate as being to its own advantage; for instance, this might be a clever but totally malevolent great white shark. Although we would not regard this as a fit subject for moral concern but rather as a menace, it is not clear that we regard it as such solely because of the threat it poses to human beings. Thus, even adding a set of 'desires' or 'preferences' to our calculating machine still does not give us what it takes to constitute a being of moral worth. This argues against the claim that 'Persons are beings with the capacity for valuing their own existence'.[9]

We are, however, getting closer to a conception of a moral agent. The contention that value 'consists in those reasons, whatever they are, that each person has for finding their own life valuable'[10] does not, however fully capture what we are after. But this formulation does embed the concept 'person' and it implies that there are aspects of a person's mental life – for instance, to do with reflection on one's own life – that are not captured by the idea of preference-ordering. The bald desire to go on living, coupled perhaps with cognitive processes apt to attain that end regardless of the impact one has on what is around one, does not seem to qualify a subject as a person. Therefore preferences, desires and interests are not equal, despite utilitarian claims to the contrary. A preference for data crunching, destroying people or pulling the wings off flies does not seem to constitute a basis for moral worth of equal weight to the desire to give and receive love from another.[11]

We could try and patch things up by taking as a basis *informed* preferences – what an agent would choose if he really knew what the alternatives before him were like – but then there is a further question as to whether the agent concerned is able to respond to the morally relevant aspects of those alternatives. It seems that there are preferences implicit within the capacity to appreciate things in the way that is required of moral agents (which is an Aristotelian thesis).[12] When we examine the preferences of certain insane people (such as the desire to eat one's own faeces or other human beings), we decide that many of them ought to be not only overridden but corrected because they are symptomatic of a deep disorder of human thought.

The argument to date suggests that difficult problems lie in wait for any moral theory which fails to analyse the content of its basic terms like preference, harm, self-consciousness and so on. But it is hard to specify most of these. Take, for instance, self-consciousness: it is unclear why a chess-playing machine that keeps track of its own moves as distinct from those made by its opponent is not self-conscious. It seems to me equally unclear whether a chimpanzee is showing self-consciousness (of the type relevant to moral concern) if it touches a dab of paint on its forehead after looking in a mirror. We therefore need to clarify just *why* self-consciousness or any other mental property, is relevant to the moral importance of a being.

(5) I can dispense with further wrangling by showing that a 'reactive attitudes' view fares rather better than its competitors in the telling 'Spanish Inquisition' case. Let us put ourselves in the moral shoes of Spanish Inquisitors. We believe that human beings have an eternal destiny and that their short span on earth prepares them for either eternal bliss or eternal agony. Thus it is clear that anything which ensures that an individual enjoys eternal bliss is good. Now imagine that certain persons are headed for eternal agony. Surely, if some temporary suffering will save them from this fate then it would be in their best interest to undergo it. If, for example, a month or so of torture will lead to an attitude change which would qualify them for eternal bliss then it would only be right to torture them, regardless of their present wishes. What is more, if there is a real danger of them slipping back into damnable attitudes, then we should kill them straight off so as to speed their eternal reward and save them from damnation or future torture with an unpredictable outcome (after all, some may be unrepentant second time around). So we have good moral reasons to employ the rack, the thumbscrew, the red hot irons and trial by burning. (The metaphysical basis is, of course, up for debate.)

Now we could dismiss this as a religious aberration of reason but we should recall that other, apparently well-reasoned arguments about the future of the human race have been used in our own century to justify genocide and similar atrocities.

I believe that the right response to such arguments is to say 'There must be something wrong with you if you can allow any argument or ideology, however rational it seems, to make you think it is right to treat another human being like that'. But *why* is this the right response?

(6) I have already argued that certain reactions, sensitivities and responses are the basis of moral judgements. We could therefore include moral judgements as part of the structure of our 'reactive attitudes'. These are judgements rather than mere feelings because the responses concerned are principled or rule-governed and can be justified.[13] In fact, the natural propensities to 'latch on', 'see what is being got at' and 'go on in the same way' that I indicated as the basis of our concept use in general all obey rules which tell us what *counts* as an instance of a given concept[14] and, in that sense, are principled or obey constraints of reason and correctness. The rules governing our concepts ramify throughout experience and order all our judgements, whether they concern colour, shape, types of object or the recognition of familiar particulars. What is more, the relevant rules are shared by others and, as we learn to think, an appreciation of the ways in which they apply certain concepts to their experience comes to order our natural reactions to, and interactions with, them.[15] Thus rational or well-grounded judgements and natural engagement between human beings as

persons are inextricably linked. It emerges that moral sensitivity – an appreciation of what matters to others and its importance – is an extension of the process of mastering communication, judgement and thought about what is happening to oneself. Where this basic and pervasive interdependence of self-thoughts/feelings with other-thoughts/feelings is lacking, moral sensitivity and depth will be vestigial (as in the case of a psychopath). Where the engagement between self and others is strong there also will moral concern be well-developed.[16]

It therefore seems that our natural reactions and our principled moral judgements are woven together in such a way that the latter are formed and given content by the former and the former are informed and articulated with our thought in general by the latter. This has important consequences for our moral reasoning in general and medical ethics in particular.

A human being has a number of relationships in which he has acquired the concepts he uses in his thinking. These concepts involve, *inter alia*, the understanding of another's suffering (conceptually linked to one's grasp of the concept 'pain'). A person also comes to appreciate the affection of others, through experiences of being nurtured and helped at points of need. He understands the wishes and needs of others because his own desires and needs are represented in terms of concepts learned through his interactions with them. Thus he has an empathy toward others just because they are human. This is both a natural tendency and a rational implication of the fact that one's system of reasons has a conceptual structure built on agreement in judgements with others. It also leaves us with two bases on which we can ground paediatric care.

A very natural (and perhaps evolutionary) response will be to take care of the young of one's own species. It is so intuitively right and continuous with qualities of affection and kindness that it is plausibly included in the foundation (in human nature) on which moral understanding is built. On this account, to harm a child or to show wanton cruelty toward another human being betrays a basic ingredient in our ability to appreciate moral judgements in general: indeed if one does not feel the force of these things one is morally destitute. Therefore we can and should say to the child-abusing father 'You must not do that!' and say it with absolute moral authority. If he retorts 'It's my child I shall do what I like with it', we can say 'If you want to do *that* then your wants do not count because in this matter you are incompetent' (note that I am considering a clear case of child battery). We recognise that a person with this kind of moral blindness is not fit to pronounce on moral questions because the reactions that are constitutive or basic to any understanding of moral concepts are defective in him. One's sensitivity to pain, distress, caring, appreciation and love are most clearly evinced when a child suffers and if they are not then one lacks something vital to one's thinking about human beings and their attributes.

We can support this appeal to the ground of the conative force of moral reasons by an independent appeal to our other reason for special regard for a child based in the idea of potentiality. An intrinsic part of human judgement is to take account of the whole of which any given feature is a part. For this reason we do not regard a cheque as being merely a piece of paper but as part of a financial transaction with its significance given that role. The totality in question, when we consider moral judgements about children, is a human life and the feature is the infant phase of such a life. Just as in the case of the cheque, we do not regard infancy in isolation. The child is part of that total form which is the focus of our moral concern and thus our attitude to the child is our attitude to a being of that type at a particularly vulnerable point. In fact, our reactions betray a very basic attitude to the being concerned – one that is uncontaminated because of the helplessness of its target by fear of reprisal.

Therefore our attitudes toward children emerge from and are given weight by a careful consideration of our nature as moral thinkers. It is, of course, from that source that moral facts arise.[17]

(7) The present account of moral reasoning, although most obviously inspired by the later Wittgenstein, also draws on Hume, Kant and Strawson.[18]

Hume places human sentiments or reactions at the heart of his account. I have argued that these emerge from our nature as needy and interrelated beings and form the basis of concepts which ground moral thought – 'pain', 'distress', 'hunger', 'love', 'sympathy' and so on. The concepts concern what matters to us and to that extent morality does draw on sentiment. It is, however, 'sound sentiment' which Hume could only specify by referring to 'the general view or survey'[19] but I have introduced a Kantian strand to the argument.

Rational beings are subjects of experience who think about the world as it is illuminated by concepts or 'rules of the understanding'. Concepts are the currency which is in use in our interactions with others where, *inter alia*, we make (potentially and essentially) shared judgements about what matters to human beings and how these things ought to figure in our practical reasoning. Where our reasoning concerns the interests of others it involves moral judgements. Moral judgements thus concern a central (interpersonal) aspect of our being as *thinking* subjects of experience. This implies that both the existence of moral properties and the force of the moral 'ought' derive directly from our reciprocity and sympathy with one another. Interpersonal reciprocity implicitly links the experiences of numerically different subjects of related kinds in virtue of the essentially shared content of the relevant concepts.[20]

Strawson makes a pivotal contribution to this position. He impresses on us the inherent generality of concepts and their univocal meanings as applied to different objects which instance them and he identifies reactive attitudes in the centre of moral judgements.[21] The first point secures the conclusion that it is implicit within the understanding of, say, 'pain' that it should have a motivating role regardless of the subject who instances it. Thus, when I recognise that someone is in pain, even though I do not feel the immediate biological force of that condition, I have a reason to intervene in the state of affairs which is producing pain. One could say that the concept 'pain' carries the implicit presumption that an occurrence of pain should motivate attempts to do something to relieve it (no matter which individual instances it). We could say that this implication was part of the 'cognitive role' of pain.

Strawson also links moral predicates to human reactions. Thus the grasp of the central moral concept 'hurt' is tied to our reactions of sympathy, concern, helping and so forth. If we lack these reactions to the condition of others we cannot even begin to grasp moral concepts because those reactions impart conative force to moral reasons. Because we have mastered these and other (holistically interwoven) concepts in and through our relationships with others, we implicitly recognise what matters to others but also feel the force of certain mental ascriptions no matter to whom they are applied.

(8) At this point, we return to medicine in general and paediatrics in particular.

Our impulse in medicine is to furnish help and comfort (using whatever technology is appropriate) to the human beings who present themselves to us. This gives professional expression to the deep-seated ethical intuitions which I have tried to characterise. These intuitions can lead to standards of dedication and professional care that many outside medicine find both idealistic and incomprehensible. It is unfortunate that this bright image is often tarnished by the stains of ambition, competition and 'filthy lucre' but nevertheless it remains as an ideal to which doctors ascribe. In paediatrics a specific aspect of our moral sense finds its expression because suffering children force ideologies and arguments back into their proper place in balanced human conduct and we are moved by deeper aspects of our moral character.

The argument that our special regard for a human infant is wrong because it is an instance of 'speciesism' can now be seen in its true colours. Rather than being an unprincipled prejudice in favour of our own species it is an expression of fundamental moral engagement with creatures whom we are coming to know as participants in a moral community. The response in question arises naturally from the fact that we include all human beings within our community of discourse and that our grasp of the concepts which inform our morality dictates that we should register what matters to them. Therefore, to suppress this deep engagement with members of our own species is to undermine one of the well-springs of moral sense and perhaps to begin to lose sight of moral facts altogether. A separate argument suggests that our moral stance toward children is an aspect of our attitude to the totality of a human life. Thus, paediatric health care workers, morally committed to the well-being of children of all ages and degrees of intelligence, express one of the most important facets of our character as moral beings.

(9) At this point we can begin to understand why it is that the death of a child, no matter how young, is such a shocking tragedy. An infant is a focus for the goodwill and concern of the family and community into which she is born. In her own immature way she reciprocates the kindness that is shown to her and responds to that goodwill with smiles, glances, utterances and gazes. As long as an infant has some capacity for love and to be loved, those who interact with him find that the warm and caring side of self meets a response which is growing and creative.[22] This response (or total pattern of responses) and the process of which it is a part culminates in the creation of a conscious, thinking human being with a unique identity. As well as having a deep and instinctive response to the infant, we thus find our most constructive, altruistic and least self-oriented tendencies enlisted in relating to a child. In a way, all that is best in oneself finds a focus in the appeal of a child. To harden oneself to this reality is a sign of moral imbecility.

When a child dies and the special relationship we have had with that child is destroyed then the tragedy involved is mitigated only by the short time in which that relationship could be shared. One parent, of deep religious convictions, remarked of this deep loss as follows: 'We know he has gone somewhere better but we so much wanted to share more of the familiar and good things we had to offer him.' To the shock of death is added, in the case of infant death, the loss of that possibility of sharing, nurturing and participating in the growth of a person. One becomes a better person by participating as a human life unfolds in response to what one has to give. These things are part of the 'bedrock' that grounds our judgements of what is good.

Any moral theory which does not exhibit this bedrock or touchstone of goodness in human character must be deficient. If we neglect what it is that creates moral value and give credence to arguments based on conceptions which do not do justice to our moral nature, our ethics is impoverished. Therefore, rather than us deriding the sentiment behind the cry 'Women and children first!', its intuitive force should alert us to a serious flaw in any ethical theory which does not endorse it.

NOTES

1 P. F. Strawson (1974) 'Freedom and resentment' in *Freedom and Resentment and Other Essays*. London: Methuen, describes these as propositional attitudes based in interpersonal relations and the reactions that we and others evince there.
2 On this argument see G. Gillett and N. Poplawski (1991) 'Ethics and embryos', *Journal of Medical Ethics* 17 2: 62–9.
3 C. S. Lewis (1970) 'Vivisection', *God in The Dock*. London: Collins; and P. Singer (1979) *Practical Ethics*. Cambridge University Press, pp. 49ff.
4 T. J. Engelhardt (1986) *The Foundations of Bioethics*. New York: Oxford University Press.
5 I have defended this view in Gillett (1992) *Representation, Meaning and Thought*. Oxford: Clarendon, especially ch. 1.
6 J. McDowell (1979) 'Virtue and reason', *Monist*, 62: 331–50.
7 Wittgenstein (1953) *Philosophical Investigations*. Oxford: Blackwells.
8 Such recognition/acquaintance outstrips, as Russell and Evans have both noted, a mere list of descriptive features.
9 J. Harris (1985) *The Value of Life*. London: Routledge and Kegan Paul, p. 25.
10 *Ibid.*, p. 16.
11 R. S. Duff and A. G. M. Campbell, 'Moral and ethical dilemmas in a special care nursery', *New England Journal of Medicine*, 289: 17.
12 Aristotle (1955) *Nicomachean Ethics*, Baltimore, MD: Penguin, Book I ch. 7.
13 Gillett (1989) 'Representations and cognitive science', *Inquiry*, 32: 261–76.
14 D. Hamlyn (1973) 'Logical and psychological aspects of learning', R. S. Peters (ed.) *The Philosophy of Education*. Oxford University Press, p. 206.
15 Gillett (1989) 'Concepts structures and meanings', *Inquiry*, 30: 101–12.
16 This thesis is defended at length in Gillett (1993) 'Ought and well-being', *Inquiry*.
17 B. Williams (1985) *Ethics and The Limits of Philosophy*. London: Fontana.
18 Peter Strawson would, I am sure, feel uncomfortable with an appellation as grand as 'moral theory' being attached to his thoughts on the subject. His modesty does not, however, undermine its intrinsic merit.
19 D. Hume (1969) *A Treatise of Human Nature* (1739) (trans. E. Mossner) Harmondsworth, Middlesex: Penguin, p. 527.
20 How close the relation must be is debatable. Wittgenstein's remark 'If a lion could talk we could not understand him' suggests that inter-translatability of language and mutual accessibility of conceptual content, which he would relate to forms of life, are important in our understanding of others and therefore in the formation of moral attitudes toward them, a point also suggested by David Wiggins (1987) in 'The person as object of science, subject of experience and

locus of moral value' in *Persons and Personality*, Peacocke and Gillett (eds.) Oxford: Blackwells.

21 Strawson (1959) *Individuals*. London: Methuen, especially ch. 3, and *Freedom and Resentment and Other Essays*. London: Methuen.

22 The capacity to love and be loved was a crucial point for Duff and Campbell and seems to be central in the 'relational potential' standard championed by Richard McCormick (e.g. in McCormick (1974) 'To save or let die: the dilemma of modern medicine', *Journal of the American Medical Association*, 229: 172–6.

11 Moral uncertainty and human embryo experimentation

Graham Oddie

Moral dilemmas can arise from uncertainty, including uncertainty of the real values involved. One interesting example of this is that of experimentation on human embryos and foetuses. If human embryos or foetuses (henceforth *embryos*) have a moral status similar to that of human persons then there will be severe constraints on what may be done to them. If embryos have a moral status similar to that of other small clusters of cells then constraints will be motivated largely by consideration for the persons into whom the embryos may develop. If the truth lies somewhere between these two extremes, the embryo having neither the full moral weight of persons, nor a completely negligible moral weight, then different kinds of constraints will be appropriate.[1] So on the face of it, in order to know what kinds of experiments, if any, we are morally justified in performing on embryos we have to know what the moral weight of the embryo is. But then an impasse threatens. For it seems implausible to many to suppose that we have settled the issue of the moral status of human embryos. It is the purpose of this chapter to show that such moral uncertainty need not make rational moral justification impossible. Section 1 develops a framework, applicable to cases of moral uncertainty, which distinguishes between what is morally right/wrong, and what is morally justified/ unjustified. In section 2 this framework is applied to the case of embryo experimentation. The upshot is that the kinds of goods which would justify performing experiments on human embryos are of the same order of value as goods which would justify comparable experiments on non-consenting persons.

1   A framework for moral uncertainty

1.1   *Three cases of uncertainty*

Case 1 Your infant son is seriously, but not terminally, ill. You have two drugs: drug **A** would effect a partial although not complete cure and this you know for sure; drug **B** is rather unusual in that its efficacy depends on chance factors at the molecular level. With your particular child it has a 2/3 chance of the right reactions taking place, thereby curing him completely, and a 1/3 chance of the wrong reactions, killing him. These are genuine physical chances, not a matter of your ignorance. But of course, even though you know all this, you cannot know in advance what the outcome will be if drug **B** is administered. Genuine chanciness implies uncertainty, while uncertainty does not necessarily imply genuine chanciness.

Case 2 Again your child is seriously, but not terminally, ill. This time you have three drugs: drug **A** as above, and drugs **C** and **D**. One of these drugs would (with chance 1) completely cure him if administered, the other would kill him (again with chance 1) if administered, but you do not know which is the killer and which the cure. To give him drug **C** would, in fact, be an act of curing him. To give him drug **D** would be to kill him. So you are uncertain which of the two acts would be the act of killing, and which the act of curing. However, you have evidence that gives you a 2/3 degree of confidence that it is drug **C** which completely cures, and a 1/3 degree of confidence that it is drug **D**.

Case 3 Your pet monkey is seriously ill. Drug **E** will cure the animal but will leave it with some discomfort and pain for the rest of its life. Drug **F** will end the animal's life painlessly. You know this, but you are unsure about the relative merits of painlessly annihilating a monkey and keeping it alive impaired. However, you have some views on the matter. You think it more likely that the monkey has a moral status akin to that of a human infant, rather than to that of a cockroach.

We are often in a position of ignorance or uncertainty about the nature and value of our actions, or of their outcomes, as cases such as these illustrate. This is obviously a problem for consequentialist moral theories. If the morally right action to perform is that with the best consequences, then to know what's right will typically require extensive knowledge not only of the value of the various possible outcomes of one's actions, but also of the causal structure of the world. In case 2 above the best action with the best consequences *in fact* is **C**, since that is the one which effects the total cure, although the agent does not know this, because he does not know the causal structure of the situation. But ignorance of causal structure is not the only generator of uncertainty. In case 1, there is uncertainty, but this time stemming not from ignorance of causal factors, but from objectively chancy factors at the micro-level. In case 3, on the other hand, you are clear about the objective chances, but uncertain about both the relative value of the monkey's life, impaired to that degree, and of painlessly ending its life.

While the problem of uncertainty is obvious for the consequentialist, deontological theories are not immune. Most kinds of actions of moral interest involve necessary conditions which go beyond the agent's behaviour, conditions which must take place if the behaviour is to constitute an act of a specified kind. Take killing and curing, for example. One cannot kill a person without him dying. One cannot cure a person without her returning to health. The dying and the returning are not part of the agent's direct behaviour. Rather the agent does something (like administering drug C or administering drug D) over which he does have more or less direct control, which has as its causal effects the dying, or the returning to health. So even if an agent can be sure that it is wrong to kill a person and right to cure him, he may find himself in a situation in which he cannot be sure which, if any, of the actions over which he has direct control will constitute an act of killing or an act of curing.

The deontologist might be tempted to respond that it is not *killing*, but rather the *intention* to kill which is morally wrong. According to this line, killings would be wrong because each and every one involves the intention to kill, and murderous intentions that do not result in deaths would be morally equivalent to those that do. Since the intention is (presumably) something of which the agent can be directly aware, and which he can (presumably) directly control, the problem of uncertainty would not arise.[2]

By declaring all the actions of moral significance to be such mental acts the deontologist may escape the problem of uncertainty – but only at enormous cost. For it seems clear that at least part of what is wrong with killing someone is that someone is killed. The wrongness of murderous intentions is at least partly to be explained by the fact that in general such intentions tend to have undesirable effects beyond the agent's own mind.

1.2   *A decision-theoretic framework*

Suppose, firstly, that the moral *rightness* or *wrongness* of an act is determined by the overall goodness or value of the act, compared with the overall goodness or value of its alternatives. For example, an act may be right only if there is no alternative option which is more valuable. Suppose, secondly, that the value of an act depends in some way on features of which you may have only limited knowledge. For example, it may be that the value of an act depends partly on the value of the actual or probable consequences of the act. Given these two assumptions you may not always know what option is the morally right one because you may not always know the precise comparative values of your options. The best you can do is to *estimate* the values of your various options on the basis of the information and beliefs you do have, and it is plausible that what you are morally *justified* in selecting is the act with the highest estimated value, by your lights.

So our two assumptions yield a natural distinction between rightness/wrongness (governed by real value), and the moral justifiability/unjustifiability (governed by estimated value in the light of your information). For example, in case 2 it would be natural to *estimate* the value of drug **A** as greater than that of either drugs **C** or **D**, since by your lights both of the latter bestow a significant probability on something of very great disvalue: killing your child.

By subordinating questions of rightness to those of value this framework may have a consequentialist ring to it. But because of its compatibility with diverse accounts of value it is applicable to an extremely broad range of moral theories, including some which it might be natural to classify as deontological. For example, it is perfectly compatible with the assigning of value or disvalue to an agent's intentions, or the particular character of the agent's performances, the kind of people we become through the performance of a certain kind of act, to the exemplification of the virtues, and so on.

But exactly how does the value of an act depend on features like its consequences? According to traditional consequentialism the value of an act is determined by how much value it would realise. But a serious problem arises because the decisive quantity, *the amount of goodness act A will/would realise*, may be undefined. Consider case 1. With the option of prescribing the chancy drug **B** there are two different possible outcomes, with very different values. If in fact the drug is administered then one could say that the value of doing so is the value of the actual outcome, either death or cure, whichever it happens to be. But suppose drug **B** is *not* administered. In that case there is simply *no answer* to the question 'How much value *would* have been realised had drug **B** been administered?' because it is not true of either outcome that it *would* have ensued if the drug had been administered. It might have produced a cure (chance 2/3) and it might have produced death (with chance 1/3).

It is here that we can take a leaf from the decision-theorist's book: the quantity which determines the value of the action is the amount of value one could (in a technical sense) *expect* the option to realise if one knew the objective chances. How much value is an action likely to realise? It is natural to measure this by its *expected* value.[3] The expected value of an action A is the weighted average of the real values of the possible outcomes of A, where each outcome is weighted by its *probability* given A.

There is thus an analytical link between probability and value: an action A has greater (expected) value the more valuable are its possible outcomes, or the more probable are its valuable outcomes.

Expected value admits of various interpretations, depending on whether the probability and value functions are either subjective or objective. Where both the probabilities and the values are objective, then we have *objective expected value* and it is this quantity which most obviously suggests itself as the determiner of an action's objective *rightness*. On this view, the morally right action is the one which would, objectively, most conduce to the good, regardless of the agent's beliefs about the good or about the causal structure of the world.

The objective chance of an outcome given A is not an epistemic matter: it is the real propensity A would bestow on that possible outcome if A were to be performed. Nor is objective value an epistemic matter. In case 1, prescribing drug B has two possible outcomes, *complete cure and death*, with respective objective chances of 2/3 and 1/3 (regardless of any particular agent's subjective probabilities) and a large value difference (regardless of any agent's desires or beliefs about value).

Let this value difference between the two outcomes (value of curing–value of killing) be c. It is only differences in value which are significant in the comparison of actions, so we can conventionally set the origin of our scale, 0, at the value of killing, and the value of curing at c. The objective expected value of administering drug **B** is the chance-weighted average of the value of the killing (0) and the value of a complete cure (c):

> objective expected value of prescribing drug **B**
> = chance of killing given that drug **B** is prescribed × value of killing + chance of a complete cure given that drug **B** is prescribed × value of a complete cure
> $= \frac{1}{3}0 + \frac{2}{3}c = \frac{2}{3}c$.

In the general case where the respective chances are p and $(1-p)$ for curing and killing, the objective expected value of administering **B** would be pc.

On the other hand a partial cure has some positive value, a value which is clearly not as great as a complete cure, but is vastly better than death: say rc, where r is a real number between 0 and 1. r measures how close (on a scale of 0 to 1) the value of a partial cure is to the value of a complete cure, and how far it is from the (dis)value of killing. Since a partial cure is much closer to a total cure than to killing, r will be rather close to 1. Prescribing drug **A** ensures (with chance 1) a partial cure. The objective expected value of prescribing drug **A** is thus just rc, and this exceeds the expected value of prescribing drug **B**, provided that r is greater than p

(= the probability that **B** will produce a cure). In case 1, if the agent ought to choose by objective value, then drug **A** is the right drug to prescribe.

Note that one might motivate the decision to prescribe drug **A** on grounds of *safety first*: that because drug **B** yields *some* risk of death, and drug **A** does not yield any, drug **A** is to be preferred. Lying behind this rationale is the principle of avoiding the worst possible outcome. (Minimise maximal possible loss.) However, the principle to which I am appealing (maximise expected value) is quite different. It tells us that a risk of death may be acceptable, *provided the chance of death is small enough to be swamped by the probability of a good outcome*: provided, that is, r is greater than p. But given that the value difference between a complete cure and death is enormously greater than that between a complete cure and a partial cure, the chance of death would have to be compensatingly very small for the risk to be worthwhile.[4]

The kind of uncertainty faced in case 1, where one drug bestows different objective chances on two possible outcomes, is analogous to the kind of uncertainty faced in case 2. But there is a difference: in case 2 what you don't know are the objective chances that your options bestow on the possible outcomes. You cannot directly apply the injunction to maximise objective expected value, since you don't know what the objective chances are. The injunction does not give you an effective selection procedure, one which is accessible to your mind. If your goal is to maximise objective value, but you don't know where maximal objective value lies, what effective selection procedure are you justified in using?

In place of employing the actual but epistemically inaccessible chances in the calculation of value, you are justified in employing your *best estimate* of these. While you may not know the objective chances, you have some information about them or at least some beliefs, and this information gives you a guide to the objective chances: possibly not a very good guide, but the best one you have. Call these estimates of the objective chances your *subjective* probabilities. If you know the actual value of outcomes, but are uncertain of the chances which your actions bestow on those outcomes, your *best estimate* of objective expected value combines your subjective probabilities with the real objective values. Subjective expected value is thus the best estimate you have of the objective expected value of your options.[5]

In case 1 substituting your subjective probabilities for the objective chances yields:

estimated value of drug =
    subjective probability of partial cure given drug × real value of
    partial cure

+ subjective probability of complete cure given drug × real value of complete cure
+ subjective probability of death given drug × real (dis)value of death

It is not hard to calculate the results of estimated value (and of objective value):

	estimated value	objective value
drug **A**	rc	rc
drug **C**	$\frac{1}{3}0 + \frac{2}{3}c = \frac{2}{3}c$	c
drug **D**	$\frac{2}{3}0 + \frac{1}{3}c = \frac{1}{3}c$	0

The estimated values are not uniformly identical to the objective expected values. But they are still your best guide to the objective values of the acts given your epistemic situation. I submit that an agent is *epistemically justified* in ranking the options according to their estimated values, and *morally justified* in choosing according to that ranking: 'morally', because of the use of real values; 'justified', because of the use of the epistemic probability measure. In case 2 drug **C** is the (objectively) right one to prescribe (as given by objective value) since it effects the complete cure – but it is not the morally justified option. The morally justified option, the one with highest estimated value in the light of your information, is drug **A**. And that is, what we would intuitively expect. Prescribing drug **C** in case 2 would be morally blameworthy, because morally unjustifiable, even though it is the objectively right thing to do.

The interesting point here is you may not only be uncertain of the objective value by virtue of uncertainty of the objective chances of outcomes. Your uncertainty may extend to the *values*. In case 3 you know what effects the drugs will have on your pet monkey, but you may well be uncertain about the values and disvalues involved. Is it really better for such an animal to live an impaired life than for that life to be painlessly ended? Perhaps there is no answer to this question, because there is no such thing as objective value. But even if there is a correct answer you don't know what it is.

I will argue that the moral uncertainty of embryo experimentation is rather like case 3. As yet we may feel we have no entirely satisfactory solution to the problem of the moral status of the embryo, and, further, this particular lacuna is not culpable ignorance. It would be, say, if by a little bit more effort on our part we could clear the matter up to the satisfaction of rational creatures apprised of all the facts accessible to us. But that seems implausible. And even if it were true, there could be other cases of non-culpable ignorance, or uncertainty, of the objective values of outcomes. Indeed, if values are objective *in some sense*, if there can be a truth of the matter as to what value we ought to attribute to outcomes, then we are almost obliged to conclude that non-culpable uncertainty of real values is a rather common phenomenon.

Given a case in which uncertainty extends to the values themselves, what choices is an agent morally justified in making? It is not enough to apply the proposal above, which employs the agent's estimates of chance together with real values of outcomes, as it stands. As in case 2, where the real chances are unknown and what is morally justified is determined by your best estimates of the chances, so in case 3 what is morally justified should be determined not by the uncertain objective values, but by your best estimates of these. If you are *rationally justified* in estimating the real value of *B* to be greater than that of *A* then you are morally justified in performing *B* rather than *A*, even if *B* is in fact objectively worse, and hence the morally wrong act.

Sense can be made of this simple idea within our decision-theoretic framework provided uncertainty of the objective values of outcomes is treated as formally tantamount to facing a number of different possible outcomes with differing objective values. Uncertainty of the real value of a particular outcome generates a set of possible (real) values of that outcome. Call these *value possibilities*. You may well have views about which value possibilities are more likely (in the purely subjective sense) than others. Idealising we can imagine that your views about value can, like your views about the natural causal facts, be represented by degrees of subjective probability.

For example, in the case of your pet monkey you may think there are two value possibilities: the first, that killing the monkey is morally equivalent to killing, say, a human infant; the second, that it is morally equivalent to killing, say, a cockroach. Suppose that you have reasons (whatever their source) for inclining to the former view (2/3 subjective probability) rather than the latter (1/3 subjective probability). It is now fairly obvious that you can estimate the value of the various options taking into account the range of value possibilities and the relative likelihood of those possibilities. In general, then, you are *morally justified in choosing to do A* just in case *A* has maximal estimated value.

There is clearly a proviso to be added here: that your ignorance or uncertainty is not culpable. There is more to be said about this, for the addition of the proviso threatens circularity. In order to specify what an agent is justified in doing, it has to be specified what he is justified in believing. A full elaboration of this account would indeed have to show that this apparent circularity is not vicious, but for our purposes we need only work with an intuitive grasp of culpable ignorance. Intuitively, an agent is culpably ignorant if he could have secured more accurate beliefs relevant to his decision problem, and he was aware of his ability to do so.

This decision-theoretic account thus has a solution to the problem of morally justifying actions in the absence of complete certainty about the objective values of outcomes, and it is to an interesting application of the framework that we now turn.

2   An application: the case of embryo experimentation

2.1   Lethal experimentation on non-consenting persons

It is widely agreed that embryos used for experimental purposes ought not to be allowed to develop into fully fledged persons. In general it is not known, in advance, quite how an experiment would affect the embryo's development. Even quite minor interventions could have dramatically detrimental effects on the person into whom the embryo would develop if allowed. Thus *The Warnock Report*, for example, recommends that no embryo used for experimental purposes be allowed to develop beyond fourteen days.[6] If this recommendation were accepted then all experimentation on embryos would be lethal, and the question of the permissibility of embryo experimentation would reduce to that of the permissibility of lethal embryo experimentation. For simplicity I will deal with the case of lethal experimentation first, and consider later whether embryo experimentation could be justified if the Warnock recommendation were rejected.

It is important to clarify the concept of a lethal experiment. An *experiment* consists in forcing an object, or system of objects, into a state it would not, or might not, otherwise enter, in order to find out what will happen to it. Experimentation thus differs from observation in that the former involves intervention and the latter does not. Experimentation also differs from therapy in that the primary end of experimentation is knowledge, whereas the primary end of therapy is healing. A *lethal experiment* is one performed on a living organism with *either* the intention that the experimental state lead directly or indirectly to the death of the organism, and it does so lead, *or* a reasonable belief that such an outcome is the likely result of the experiment, and it is.

Lethal experiments on non-consenting persons are almost universally thought to be seriously wrong. Moreover, the wrongness of such experiments is not thought to consist solely in their lethality. Many killings which are wrong do not seem as wrong as lethal experiments. Some, at least, of the carnage of World War Two was wrong, and judged to be so. But the lethal experiments routinely performed by Joseph Mengele on non-consenting persons were widely judged to be of a different order of wrongness altogether. There will be different explanations of this judgement on different moral theories, but it is not necessary here to adjudicate between them. This judgement on lethal experiments can be taken here as a *prima facie* moral datum which any moral theory must attempt to accommodate. The judgement could be overturned (corrected) by an otherwise extremely powerful and attractive moral theory but, other things being equal, a moral theory which delivers this judgement is to be preferred to one which does not.

A programme of lethal experiments on non-consenting persons might well be a promising source of very valuable information. Such information might have intrinsic scientific value (if indeed information has intrinsic value), or it might yield medical procedures which would benefit many other people enormously. The fact is, however, that such programmes are not usually put forward for research funds. Or, if they are, they are turned down. Or, if they are not turned down, the public does not get to hear about them. Or, if the public does get to hear about them, there is general moral outrage.[7] An excellent decision-theoretic explanation for this collection of facts is that the disvalue of a programme of lethal experiments on non-consenting persons is judged to outweigh heavily the value of the kinds of goods which such a programme might be expected to yield.[8] There may be possible circumstances which would justify a programme of such experiments, and it may be that in such circumstances people would agree that they were justified, even if no one were willing to volunteer. For example, they might be justified if it appeared likely that the only alternative was the extinction of the human race, or its survival under totally unacceptable conditions. But all that is required for our purposes here is that such circumstances do not often turn up.[9]

2.2   *The moral status of the embryo*

If the abortion debate has made one thing clear it is the extraordinary difficulty of achieving some kind of rational consensus on the moral status of human embryos. Note that while the issues of abortion and experimentation both centre on the problem of the embryo's moral status it should not be assumed that positions on abortion will simply coincide with positions on embryo experimentation. Those who think that abortion is morally permissible are not compelled to accept the permissibility of lethal experimentation. Firstly, embryos which are used for experimental purposes will normally be sustained in an artificial environment, outside the womb, and so the question of a woman's rights with respect to her own body need not enter the picture.[10] Secondly, if section 1 is on the right lines, lethal experiments can reasonably be regarded as worse than ordinary killings. It can be permissible (or obligatory) to kill a being without it being permissible (or obligatory) to lethally experiment on it. Thus we can afford to sideline the problem of the moral justifiability of abortion here, though we cannot afford to ignore whatever that debate has taught us about the moral status of the embryo.

Wertheimer argued, in 'Understanding the abortion argument' that the prospects for a satisfactory, rational resolution of the issue of the embryo's moral status were poor, and the subsequent development of the debate is evidence in favour of Wertheimer's claim.[11] There is no doubt that the issues are much clearer now than they were twenty years ago. For example, we now know not to confuse the concept of a human being with that of a person, or that of a human person.[12] It is fairly well established that purely biological characteristics are not morally relevant.[13] Much excellent work has been done to clarify the moral relevance of potential personhood. But despite these significant gains in understanding, the debate seems not to have reached a satisfactory conclusion, let alone any kind of consensus.

There will, of course, be those on both sides of the debate who will disagree strongly with this claim. Instead of attempting to convince them by rehearsing the old arguments, or attempting to construct new arguments for either side, I will take Wertheimer's claim as a premise, and see what follows from it. Those who are reluctant to embrace fully the consequences of either of the rival positions must acknowledge that we are uncertain about the moral status of the embryo. Moreover, if Wertheimer is right, this ignorance does not stem from a failure to search thoroughly for the truth, but from the nature of the problem. What are we justified in doing with embryos given an acknowledgement of that uncertainty?

The application of the decision-theoretic framework to the case of lethal embryo experimentation will be developed in three stages, at each stage relaxing an important simplifying assumption.

2.3   *The first version: two possibilities for moral weight*

The basic structure of the argument is simple. We face a choice between experimenting on embryos and not experimenting. Simplifying, either the embryo does have the same moral status as a person or it has no moral weight at all. (That the embryo has the same moral weight as a person is not, of course, equivalent to saying that it *is* a person.) This generates four possibilities:

	Embryo has moral weight of person	Embryo has no moral weight
Experiment	First possibility	Second possibility
Don't experiment	Third possibility	Fourth possibility

On the assumption most favourable to experimentation, experimenting will deliver valuable goods not otherwise obtainable. Let us agglomerate these and dub them, *the good*: of value g. So this good is obtained in both the first and second possibilities, but not in the third and fourth. On the other hand, by experimenting there is the possibility of something decidedly lacking in value: lethally experimenting on a being with the same moral weight as a person. Call this, *the evil*: of value l. It is crucial to note that the evil is *equivalent to the evil of lethally experimenting on a non-consenting person*. This evil arises only given *both* that we experiment *and* that embryos have the same moral weight as persons: the first possibility. So the good arises only in possibilities one and two, and the evil only in possibility one. Let us assume that the good and the evil are commensurable and tradable. In other words, the value of the first possibility is the sum of the good and the evil, $g - l$, whereas the value of the second possibility is just the good alone: g. It is only value differences that count in ranking possibilities and, since the third and fourth possibilities involve neither the good nor the evil, we can set the value of both at 0. Thus our table of value looks like this:

	Embryo has moral weight of person	Embryo has no moral weight
Experiment	$g - l$	g
Don't experiment	0	0

The salient feature of this table is that, provided the argument of section 2.1 is right, it is strongly asymmetrical. In normal cases l will be very large in comparison with g. It is this asymmetry which does most of the work in what ensues.

To rank the two possible courses of actions we compare their subjective expected values. Let p be one's subjective probability that the embryo has moral weight, and $(1 - p)$ the probability that it does not. Then the expected value of experimenting is:

probability of the first possibility given experimentation × value of the first possibility

+ probability of the second possibility given experimentation × value of the second possibility

$= p(g - l) + (1 - p)g$

$= g - pl$
$=$ (value of the good) minus (the disvalue of the evil $\times$ probability of the embryo having moral weight).

The expected value of not experimenting is just 0 ($= p0 + (1-p)0$). So for experimentation to be preferable, the expected value of experimenting must be greater than that of not experimenting. And that will hold just in case g is greater than pl. That is, the value of the good must be greater than the disvalue of the evil $\times$ probability of the embryo having moral weight.

We are making a number of simplifying assumptions which favour the case for experimentation. Firstly, the costs in terms of resources which such experiments must involve are ignored. Secondly, even if embryos do have the same moral status as persons we assume that the goods obtained by experimenting retain their value despite their etiology. (This may seem innocuous, but it could easily be challenged. Consider the moral indignation when it was revealed a number of years ago that scientists were using data Mengele had derived from his lethal experiments on non-consenting persons.) Thirdly, it is certain that experimenting will yield the good and that failing to experiment will deprive us of the good.

I have argued (section 2.1) that the magnitude of the evil at issue (lethally experimenting on non-consenting persons) is much greater than that of the good we could hope to derive thereby. So for the inequality to hold the probability of the embryo having moral weight must be vanishingly small. But given uncertainty as to the embryo's moral weight (section 2.2) that is false.

We can approach the result in another way without relying on the conclusion of section 2.1. For lethal experimentation on non-consenting persons (disvalue $= l$) to be justified by the certain prospect of, say, a cure for leukemia (value $= g$), we would have to have $g > l$. But given our ignorance of the moral status of the embryo (say, $p = 1/2$) to justify lethal experimentation on embryos we would have to have: $2g > l$. But then g (the value of the cure) and l (the disvalue of lethal experimentation) are not of a different order of magnitude: g is within reach of l. Suppose that the value of a cure for leukemia is roughly that of a cure for AIDS, and the value of having both is roughly twice that of having one such cure. Then if we judge it justifiable to experiment lethally on embryos to obtain one of these cures, the certitude of both cures would justify a programme of lethal experimentation on non-consenting persons. Looked at in this way the argument shows that a positive attitude to embryo experimentation calls for a rather drastic revision in our judgement of the relative merits of lethally experimenting on non-consenting persons.[14]

2.4 *The second version: continuity of moral weight and pure agnosticism*

Beings do not fall into just two categories, those with the full moral weight of persons, and those with zero moral weight. Rather, moral weight is (at least in principle) a continuous magnitude.[15] The first version of the argument is thus simplified, but the simplification is not vicious.

We may assume that the moral weight of the embryo (w), compared with that of a human person, lies between 0 and 1 (inclusive), and that the disvalue of lethally experimenting on embryos is wl. The moral weight of the embryo is thus fixed by the intrinsic disvalue of lethally experimenting on embryos compared with the intrinsic disvalue of lethally experimenting on non-consenting persons. It is the ratio of the former to the latter. We thus rule out the possibility that embryos are worth more than ordinary human persons ($w > 1$) and the possibility that lethally experimenting on them could be *intrinsically* valuable ($w < 0$). We are now dealing with a continuous magnitude, and the discrete probability assignment to the two value possibilities gives way to a probability density over the possible values of the magnitude w. Given your particular probability density we can calculate the *expectation* of w (E_w) which is, roughly speaking, what you could expect w to be, given your particular beliefs. We could call E_w the embryo's *estimated* moral weight, and it turns out that estimated moral weight plays exactly the same role in this second version as does p (the probability that the embryo has the full moral weight of a person) in the first version. That is to say, it is easy to show that experimentation is justifiably preferred to the alternative just in case $E_w < g/l$.

Pure agnosticism over the precise location of the value of w in the unit interval is tantamount to a principle of indifference: that the probability distribution over the possible weights is perfectly even. This yields the result that E_w, the estimated moral weight of the embryo, is $1/2$. Thus the assumption of pure agnosticism about the embryo's moral weight, yields precisely the same result as an equal probability assignment to the two extremes of the spectrum. As before experimentation is morally justifiable just in case: $2g > l$.

2.5 *The third version: relaxing agnosticism*

Pure agnostics thus have grounds for resisting lethal embryo experimentation comparable to the grounds (if any) they have for resisting lethal experimentation on non-consenting persons. While many would agree with the pure agnostic that we do not known for certain what the moral weight of the embryo is, they would claim that the balance of probabilities is definitely in favour of a low weight rather than a high weight. They might claim that the arguments against a high weighting are not absolutely compelling but that they are nevertheless more powerful than the opposing arguments. So we may be relatively confident that the moral weight of the embryo is small rather than large.

The assumption of relative confidence could be spelt out in a number of ways. It would have to entail that the estimated moral weight of the embryo is less than $1/2$. But even quite a small estimated weight, say $1/10$, would still generate a moral problem for experimentation. It would entail that if lethal experimentation on embryos is morally justified to obtain a good g, then lethal experimentation on non-consenting persons is justified to obtain goods ten times the value of g.[16]

2.6   Non-lethal experimentation

An advocate of embryo experimentation might well take this argument to be a *reductio* of *The Warnock Report*'s recommendation that embryo experimentation be lethal. The response might be that embryos used for experimental purposes ought to be given a reasonable chance to survive and develop. But suppose that a certain kind of experiment on an embryo is advocated. The point of the experiment is to find out what will happen to the embryo when it is forced into the experimental state. If we knew in advance what would happen to the embryo there would be no point in subjecting it to the experiment. Thus if the experiment is to be of value we would have to be reasonably ignorant, in advance, of the likely effects on the embryo of the experimental state. Thus any such experiment would involve a risk of harm, possibly a considerable one, to the person into whom the embryo would develop. Even if we put to one side the issue of the embryo's moral status, non-lethal experimentation would be subject to the same constraints appropriate to experimentation on non-consenting persons. Thus non-lethal experimentation on human embryos is likewise justified only if the goods to be obtained are comparable to those which would justify similarly risky experiments on non-consenting persons.

3   Implications

The argument establishes that, given value uncertainty, it is morally justified to perform lethal (or risky) experiments on embryos only if it is morally justified to perform lethal (or risky) experiments on non-consenting persons to obtain comparable goods. Apart from that of value uncertainty, the assumptions of the final version of the argument are all either relatively uncontroversial or they favour embryo experimentation.

Of course, any argument can be regarded as a challenge to its premises. Thus those committed to the justifiability of experimentation may well take this to establish what they have assumed all along: that embryos are of negligible moral weight. Or they may even begin to suspect that the blanket proscription against lethal experimentation on non-consenting persons is itself unjustified. But what the argument certainly shows is that the strongly asymmetrical value structure of this particular moral dilemma imposes the onus of proof very heavily on one side of the debate. Moderate agnostics on the question are forced to take sides with those who claim that embryos have the same moral status as human persons. Thus even if experimentation on human embryos happens to be morally *right*, it will be difficult to justify morally. And, of course, an analogous conclusion will apply to any moral problem in which the possible value outcomes exhibit the same strong asymmetry.

ACKNOWLEDGEMENTS

Earlier versions of this chapter were read at seminars at Otago University and Hebrew University and at a meeting of the British Society for the Philosophy of Science in London. I would like to thank all of those who have made comments and criticisms: particularly Grant Gillett, Frank Jackson, Hugh Mellor, Roy Perrett and Philip Pettit.

NOTES

1 *The Warnock Report* (1984); that is, the *Report of the Committee of Inquiry into Human Fertilisation and Embryology.* (London: Her Majesty's Stationery Office), endorses an intermediate position of this kind. On the basis of this intermediate status the report argues (pp. 64–5) that 'embryo research should not be totally prohibited. We do not want to see a situation in which human embryos are frivolously or unnecessarily used in research ...', but '... continued research is essential, if advances in treatment and medical knowledge are to combine.'

2 This is one interpretation of Kant's theory of the good will: see 'The good will and its results' in *Groundwork of the Metaphysics of Morals* edn H. J. Paton (1972) *The Moral Law* (London: Hutchinson) p. 60.

3 See G. Oddie and P. Milne (forthcoming) 'Act and value: expectations and the representability of moral theories' in *Theoria* for the thesis that acts should be evaluated by the expected value of the various possible outcomes with which they are compatible.

4 A thorough application of the safety first principle would make our lives intolerable. See J. C. Harsanyi (1976) 'Can the maximin principle serve as a basis for morality? A critique of John Rawl's theory', in *Essays on Ethics, Social Behaviour, and Scientific Explanation* (Dordrecht: Reidel) p. 37ff.

5 See P. Menzies and G. Oddie (1992) 'An objectivist's guide to subjective value'

in *Ethics* 102: 3 pp. 512–33 for a full defense of this position. This draws on earlier work by Frank Jackson (1986) in 'A probabilistic approach to moral responsibility' *Proceedings of the Seventh International Congress of Logic, Methodology, and Philosophy of Science*, R. Barcan Marcus *et al.* (eds.) (Amsterdam: North-Holland Publishing Co.).

6 *The Warnock Report* (1984) p. 66.

7 J. Katz's (1972) *Experimentation with Human Beings* (New York: Russell Sage Foundation) is a fascinating compendium of material on the subject. Particularly interesting in this connection is the Jewish Chronic Diseases Hospital Case (1963) in which chronically (though not terminally) ill patients were, without their informed consent, injected with live cancer cells to test their immunological response. (Opinion is divided over whether this could have induced a serious malignancy.) These experiments were not lethal according to our definition (none of the patients died as a result of them, and probably none was intended to die) but they certainly bear a resemblance to lethal experiments, and the episode, as recorded in the documents assembled by Katz, does bear out our four-fold 'thesis' about such experiments. (1) The programme was not submitted for proper scrutiny by the appropriate authorities before it was implemented. (2) If it had been it seems it would have been rejected. (3) Had it not been for a patient's complaint the episode might never have been exposed. (4) And once it was exposed public reaction against it was strong.

8 One way of accommodating such a judgement is sketched by A. Sen (1982) in his 'Rights and agency', *Philosophy and Public Affairs*, 11, no. 1, pp. 3–39. A 'goal rights system' is one in which 'fulfilment and non-realisation of rights are included among the goals, incorporated in the evaluation of states of affairs, and then applied to the choice of actions through consequential links'. (p. 13) A much more systematic framework which shows that this is always theoretically possible is presented in Oddie and Milne (forthcoming).

9 A non-consequentialist might give a different explanation. For example, it might be argued that persons have a *right* not to be lethally experimented upon no matter what goods might be derived from such experiments. This can be assimilated to the decision-theoretic explanation by assigning a disvalue to lethal experiments which is so large that no feasible amassing of the sorts of goods which could be derived from such experiments could ever compensate. See Oddie and Milne (forthcoming) for the details.

10 J. J. Thomson (1971) has argued in 'A defense of abortion', *Philosophy and Public Affairs*, 1, no. 1, pp. 47–66 that even if the foetus (or the embryo) has the full moral weight of a person it is not always wrong to abort it. However, Thomson acknowledges that her argument shows only that the woman has the right to dislodge the foetus or embryo, not the right to ensure its death, let alone the right to perform lethal experiments on it. A Thomson-type argument could not establish the legitimacy of lethal experimentation on doomed foetuses or embryos, unless we add, as a general principle, that a doomed organism is fair game for lethal experimenters. And that, in general, is clearly unacceptable.

11 R. Wertheimer, (1971) 'Understanding the abortion argument', *Philosophy and Public Affairs* 1, no. 1, pp. 67–95.

12 For a clear account of the distinction and a survey of the arguments see M. Tooley (1983) *Abortion and Infanticide* (Oxford University Press), pp. 50–86.

13 *Ibid.*, pp. 61–77.

14 A related argument has been put forward by Lachlan Chipman in a short article 'By whom begot: IVF, law making and moral uncertainty', *Quadrant*, 28, no. 9, pp. 16–17. However, Chipman inclines to the *safety first* principle of minimising maximal loss. Consider, 'Killing people whose lives might be saved is so abhorrent, that the fact that there is a chance, even a remote chance, that our conduct would produce that result is enough to make it unacceptable'. (p. 17) What is all important is the *degree* of remoteness of the chance. Perhaps there is a remote (*very* remote) chance that potatoes have the same moral weight as persons. This should not stop us eating chips, for the simple reason that the chance is so *very* remote, and this is precisely what the principle of expected value delivers. (This also answers an attack by Wertheimer (1971) 'Understanding the abortion argument', *Philosophy and Public Affairs* 1, no. 1, p. 76, on a simple minded version of the argument from uncertainty.)

15 An interesting discussion of the idea that the physiological continuity from blastocyst to adult human yields some kind of continuity of moral weight is to be found in N. Poplawski and G. Gillett (1991) 'Ethics and embryos', *The Journal of Medical Ethics* June. Poplawski and Gillett argue that the value which attaches to a human life as a temporal whole must also attach (at least partly) to its temporal stages, and hence even to the early stages of such a life. This is compatible with (although does not entail) the possibility that the embryo has a significant value, albeit not the same value as a fully functioning person.

16 Also, if the estimated moral weight of the embryo/foetus increases with its age we get the intuitively correct result that the difficulty of justification also increases with age.

12 Morality: invention or discovery?

James O. Urmson

In this chapter I propose to discuss in a very general and, no doubt, superficial way an ancient and fundamental question in moral philosophy and then indicate how it is relevant to our approach to practical problems, some of which concern us all, and some of which are of primary importance to the medical profession.

The ancient and fundamental question is how we arrive at our moral code. Is the moral code something that we discover by pure thought to be necessarily binding, perhaps somewhat similarly to the way in which by pure thought we can see the necessity of mathematical truths? If so, are those who cannot see the correctness of the moral code we uphold to be thought of as rather like people who are bad at arithmetic or untrained in arithmetic? Or are we to think of moral truths as more like the findings of empirical science? Is it, for example, the case that we discover, by introspection or by inspection of our neighbours, that human beings are so framed that they (almost invariably) favour some types of behaviour and disfavour others rather as they (almost invariably) like and dislike the same basic flavours? Or are we to think of our moral code as rather like the highway code, or at least like the positive laws made by governments, the invention of human beings, like the wheel and the spade? On the first two of these views we may say that moral codes are discovered; the world, or human beings, being as they are, morality is a feature of the landscape to which we must adapt ourselves. On the third view they are inventions; man invents moral codes because, for whatever reason, he finds it desirable to do so. This last view does not suggest that morality is unimportant or indifferent; there are desirable and undesirable inventions, desirable and undesirable legislation and good and bad highway codes.

These three views seem to cover most of the theories put forward by philosophers, since, as here stated, all are very general and admit of many varieties within them. The first covers most varieties of objectivism, including the Thomistic view of morality as discerned by natural reason, Kantianism, intuitionism that claims simply to see the validity of a variety of moral precepts and, at any rate, a utilitarianism based, like Moore's, on

162

a claim to see the basic principle of utilitarianism as self-evident. The second covers the many varieties of moral sense theories, such as those of Hutcheson and Hume, but need not follow the moral sense view except in general character. The third covers a wide variety of views, from the Calvinistic view that the moral code is the legislation of God, to the Marxist theory that moral codes are a weapon of a dominant class in class warfare, as well as the intermediate view that mankind adopts a moral code because it needs one, as it adopts most other inventions.

If we choose suitable examples it is quite easy to see the attraction of all three types of view. Thus, it is very natural to say that the infliction of gratuitous pain on sentient creatures is self-evidently wrong; when, if ever, the infliction of pain can be justified may be difficult to determine, but it seems obvious that it needs justification. To defend the infliction of gratuitous pain is to claim that its infliction needs no justification as such, just as going for a walk needs no justification as such (the point of adding 'as such' is that anything can be rendered wrong by the circumstances; a doctor who left a critically ill patient in order to take a walk would, no doubt, be misbehaving). We might describe anyone who does not see the wrongness of inflicting gratuitous pain as being morally blind, as a moral imbecile. We may argue seriously about the rights and wrongs of vivisection, regarding our opponent as rational and as having a case to answer, whatever view we ourselves take; but one who defended it by saying 'What's wrong with inflicting pain, anyway?' would seem to be beyond the reach of rational discourse. To G. E. Moore it seemed equally self-evident that the action which among those possible would produce the maximum net good must always be right; to many others the rightness of respect for life, gratitude and many other things has seemed equally self-evident.

It is this self-evidence, the notion that those who disagree must be moral imbeciles and beyond the reach of rational discourse, that makes us tend to see morality as a set of rational truths, akin to those of mathematics. No empirical belief is irrational in this way. It may be irrational to continue to believe that the earth is flat in the face of the available evidence, for to make correct inferences is part of rationality. But the belief that the earth is flat is in itself one that very many rational men held in former times. By contrast, the wrongness of the gratuitous infliction of pain seems to need no evidence. Mathematicians have devised calculi in which $2+2=4$ is proved, but it needs no proof and was certainly known before the invention of these calculi; in the same way this moral truth seems to need no proof, even if moral calculi could be devised in which it was a theorem. Just as we should think anyone who denied that $2+2=4$, or even denied its evidence, was, mathematically, an imbecile, so with some basic moral truths.

Not all philosophers have been able to accept the view stated above. Among those who reject it are some who would agree that such basic moral precepts as that prohibiting the gratuitous infliction of pain were indeed obvious and acceptable to all (normal) persons, but who would reject the mathematical analogy and, in general, the appeal to pure reason. Thus David Hume held that reason alone could determine only matters of fact, whether in the pure or in the empirical sciences or in everyday life; but no matter of fact was in itself capable of influencing conduct. Thus the knowledge that the glass that I hold in my hand contains poison will not on its own influence me to abstain from drinking its contents; for that the will or desire to remain alive is also necessary. Since the belief that the gratuitous infliction of pain is wrong does most certainly influence the believer's conduct it cannot be a deliverance of reason. It must be rather an expression of the will and desires of the believer. It is a prescription, a programme, a recommendation, rather than a truth discerned by pure reason or experiment.

So Hume, and those who think with him, have to reject our first view of morality. But they would, none the less, agree that certain basic moral truths require universal acceptance. In Hume's version the argument runs roughly as follows: the basic elements in human nature are virtually identical in almost all human beings; with the exception of a few people regarded as abnormal we see things in the same colours, find the same things sweet or bitter, loud or soft, painful or pleasant, cold or hot. Among these basic facts about human nature is the fact that we (almost) all find the gratuitous infliction of pain hateful and, for example, gratitude for benefits agreeable. This universal truth about human nature is the central element in the explanation why we find shared moral codes in the world and why we all assent to the prohibition of gratuitious infliction of pain and accept the demand for gratitude for benefits received as obvious. We cannot but assent to such moral injunctions; we do not choose them or invent them; unlike most of our choices they are not within our control. We cannot decide to accept or to reject such injunctions, any more than we can decide whether to find tastes sweet or bitter.

So both the views outlined agree that it would be abnormal not to accept these basic injunctions. But for the first view the abnormality is one of intelligence, a type of irrationality, for the second it is more like a defect of hearing or one of the other senses. Moral blindness will have some likeness to colour-blindness. But whereas colour-blindness leads to abnormal judgements of fact, moral blindness leads to abnormal approval and disapproval. There is, moreover, another important difference between these disabilities of the five senses and moral blindness. The blind and the deaf are harmed rather than harmful; it is they who suffer not their fellows. But the morally blind will act in a way contrary to the interests of others and in ways that are repugnant to them: they are harmful; they damage the maintenance of a society such as suits the needs and desires of their fellows. Moral blindness is incomparably more important than the other abnormalities with which it may in some respects be compared.

I have described this second theory with reference to Hume, though the reader should be warned, if it be necessary, that it would be partial, over-simplified, and so inaccurate as a presentation of Hume's views. We must now go on to consider why some have rejected both the views outlined and have claimed that morality is a human invention.

There is, of course, no one single answer to this question, but probably the consideration which has weighed most commonly and most heavily with objectors to the first two views is that, so far from there being one single common moral code acceptable to all rational beings, or to all who share in human nature, quite rational human beings all over the world have accepted in all sincerity quite different moral codes. Thus these two views presuppose and explain a purely imaginary situation. Those who accept them presumably project the relatively close agreement on morality at their place and in their time on to the universe and eternity.

The discovery of the variety in morals can lead, and has led, to moral scepticism. Thus, when the ancient Greeks began to be familiar with the moral customs of their neighbours, Thrasymachus, according to Plato in his *Republic*, concluded that morality was an invention of the powerful to keep the rest in subjection and Glaucon stated the case for the equally sceptical, but incompatible, view that it was the invention of the many weak to fetter the strong. These are sceptical views, which led adventurous thinkers like Callias in Plato's *Gorgias* to the view that one should be moral when one must and immoral when one can.

But the view that moral codes are human inventions does not obviously and at once lead to a sceptical rejection of them. Highway codes are very clearly human inventions, but are none the less acceptable for that. If it be said, falsely, that so long as we have a highway code it is indifferent which we have, it is at least clear that every civil society needs a code of man-made law and that such codes may certainly be good or bad. So the view that our moral code is a man-made invention is not inherently cynical, sceptical or luke-warm. It is possible for a holder of this view to regard morality as of prime importance. He may think that without such a code neither he nor anyone else could achieve a life worth living.

But how accurate is the claim that moral codes vary greatly from time to time and place to place? This is clearly a question to which a full answer would require a fat tome written in collaboration by a team of philosophers, anthropologists, sociologists and, no doubt, others. But a few doubting queries are all that I am capable of.

(1) We must distinguish between two moral codes differing in content and those differing in scope. Thus respect for human life may be common to societies that recognise only the family, or the village, or the tribe, or white men, or some other group, as belonging to them and thus within the protection of morality. The ancient Greeks did not think of non-Greeks, known collectively as barbarians, as being in their social group and did not acknowledge all the moral constraints on behaviour towards them that were required towards fellow-Greeks. Of old the Australians went out shooting aborigines for sport, but punished the murder of white Australians with death, and parallels to this can be found in all societies, both in the past and in the present. It still remains that few humans think of non-humans as members, or full members, of their society, and that the obligation to respect life applies to them in the same way as to human animals. But it is hard to imagine any stable society in which the members were not regarded as having a right to some degree of security, whatever complications are introduced by human sacrifice and the like.

(2) Some explicitly different moral precepts may be found to serve implicitly the same moral function. Thus if one were to find monogamy to be the moral norm in one society where adult members of the two sexes were approximately equal in numbers and polygamy the moral norm in another where, for some such reason as endemic tribal warfare, there was a severe shortage of adult males, it might be thought that in each case the norm was designed to ensure general sexual satisfaction, maintenance of numbers and the like. Similarly, some part of the general easing of moral condemnation of sexual promiscuity in our time is surely explained by the view that the true moral objection was to irresponsible parenthood, which could now be avoided by methods of birth control, though one would be naive to think that this was the whole story. Again, it is no doubt desirable that children should feel a moral obligation of care towards aged parents in a society like ours; but in a nomadic society in which a young woman may marry into a family which loses contact with her parents some modification of that obligation is surely required.

(3) Those who deny that morality is a man-made invention are not so profoundly ignorant as to be unaware that there are variations in historically accepted moral codes. They are also aware that people have claimed to square the circle and to find finite numerical values for *pi*, but have not been led to suppose that mathematics is arbitrary. They believe that people's moral perception has been distorted by superstition, ignorance and stupidity, and that public codes have been further influenced by

greed, hypocrisy and fraud. If, they hold, moral truth is to be discovered, it does not follow that every society will succesfully discover it. There is true morality and mistaken morality. The doctrine of progress has been historically linked with a belief that morality, like science, is continually approaching nearer to truth. Revealed religions normally include the true morality as part of what has been revealed to the otherwise misguided. Whether these claims are to be accepted may be doubted; but clearly the mere fact of divergence in moral beliefs, to the extent that it occurs, is surely not a refutation of their views.

(4) Once we make allowance for the points already noticed, we may be willing to agree that at least many of the apparent differences between the moral codes accepted at different times and in different places are morally neutral and reflect the different needs and circumstances of different societies; at least some differences of substance, such as the admission or non-admission of such punishments as hanging, drawing and quartering may well be thought to represent a genuine advance in moral standards. There seem to be some basic norms of behaviour without which a society could scarcely continue, and others without which it could scarcely flourish. I have in mind such things as security of life and property, promise-keeping, truth-telling. That there are local variants of such matters is clear; that any society should not have recognised them in some form seems inconceivable. It is notorious that even at more rarified levels it is hard to find any teaching of prophet, saint or guru that has not been anticipated or paralleled by another in entire independence; we might expect still more uniformity in matters which seem to be basic to any community.

We can, of course, be more eclectic in our opinions. Faced with the great debate in ancient Greece whether laws and customs were natural (*phusei*) or man-made and thus conventional (*thesei*), Aristotle said that some were one and some the other. He had not in mind the mere fact that laws were passed by governments. What was already a natural law might be enshrined in government legislation. The natural was what was universally acknowledged, the man-made was what was merely local. It was, he thought, too improbable to believe that all societies would have independently accepted certain basic precepts if they were arbitrary.

Hume also, whom we have used to illustrate the view that our moral beliefs were determined by human nature and not by choice, held that in addition to what he called natural virtues there were what he called artificial virtues. It was, he thought, inevitable in human nature to be pleased by the sight of gratitude and kindness. But justice could be very displeasing; if one man borrows from another, meets with financial catastrophe, and can only repay the debt, not seriously needed by the creditor, by depriving his wife and children of their basic needs, the repayment, Hume thought, is repugnant in the way that kindness is pleasing, but it is just. Men in a complex society, he held, need to create the artificial virtue of justice because without it, trade, commerce and other complex dealings would be impossible. Hume hastens to add that by calling justice artificial he is not belittling it, and that in a way it is natural: 'mankind is an inventive species; and where an invention is obvious and absolutely necessary, it may properly be said to be natural as anything that proceeds immediately from original principles . . . Though the rules of justice are *artificial*, they are not arbitrary' (Hume, 1911, *Treatise of Human Nature*, Everyman edn. Vol. II, London: J. M. Dent Ltd, pp. 184ff.).

But let us now leave this rather rarified discussion and turn to more practical implications and considerations.

(1) In the first place, it is surely clear that there are some basic moral precepts that nobody seriously doubts or debates. I have in mind such requirements as respect for life, liberty and property, promise-keeping and truth-telling. This holds whether they be discoveries or necessary inventions. It is no doubt proper that as philosophers we should ask why we accept such basic and obvious moral precepts, just as we ask as philosophers why we believe that chairs and tables and other people exist; but as practical persons we cannot seriously doubt their validity.

(2) But these basic precepts are not a sufficient guide to conduct for at least two reasons:

(a) such precepts need interpretation and amplification in order to be applied to many concrete situations. Thus, which of a man's possessions are his rightful property? Possession is said to be nine points of the law, but it is not ten-tenths of the moral law. Are war and capital punishment compatible with respect for life? Some will claim that the answer is obvious, but they will not agree about which answer that is. Is a doctor never justified in lying to a patient, and, if ever, when? Are there no circumstances in which a promise may be broken, and if there are, what are they? This difficulty in applying basic moral precepts has always been recognised and the attempt to answer them has been called traditionally casuistry (which should not be a pejorative term, for casuistry in morals is as necessary and inevitable as is legal argument about the application of positive law).

(b) there are moral problems where such basic precepts, however refined and elaborated by casuistry, seem to go but a minimal distance towards solving our problems. A claim to solve such problems as when, if ever, surrogate motherhood and AID are justified, whether the possession of nuclear weapons is justified, whether battery chicken farming is justified, and so many others by any appeal to some generally acknowledged basic principle must be fraudulent. Part of the difficulty is no doubt the dispassionate collection of all the relevant facts and their clear presentation. No doubt the basic moral precepts remain relevant as limiting the range of possible solutions. But it seems inevitable that we must sit down and devise for ourselves a code of behaviour. There is none ready-made. Philosophers often talk as though there were readily available pre-existing moral precepts in the light of which each moral issue was to be determined, however novel and however complicated. But this is surely a myth.

Given this situation, it is useless for those involved to appeal to any natural authority to answer their questions. If they accept a supernatural authority as capable of answering them, well and good. If not, they have to answer the questions themselves. I have heard respected medical men reproach moral philosophers with not providing a solution to the problems, but this is a misunderstanding of what moral philosophers can do. Certainly they have no special moral insight not found in other men. They can attempt to state accurately and clearly the relevant facts known to them, they can attempt to argue dispassionately and rigorously, they can make distinctions that might be overlooked, but they cannot pontificate, or, rather, when they do they are exceeding their authority. Moral philosophers can, indeed, and should attempt to help. I believe that some of the many philosophical writings on abortion, for example, have helped significantly to make the issues clear. I hope and believe, therefore, that it is useful for moral philosophers, by which I mean not just professionals but all who are willing to make the effort to think clearly and dispassionately at a fairly high level of generality, to sit in, as it were, on the discussion of all these complex issues. To take a concrete example, I think it was wise to ask Mary Warnock, a moral philosopher, to chair the Warnock Committee. But philosophers must sit in as sharers in a search, not as authorities.

A typical case where clear, philosophical thought, whether by professional philosophers, the medical profession, lawmakers or others, is necessary might be the question of the time at which a life may be said to begin. It is clearly an issue where knowledge of the relevant scientific facts is essential; it is clear that some sort of moral judgement is involved. But we also need to ask such conceptual questions as: what do we mean by 'living organism'?; do we mean the same by 'living organism' as we mean by 'living person'?; if we do not mean the same by these two expressions, what do we mean by 'living person'? We shall also have to ask such questions as: does the concept of a living person include the concept of a living human embryo?, and we shall have to face the fact that there is no pre-existing answer to such a question that we merely have to discover. The scope of concepts is determined by linguistic use, and language here gives us no clear answer; the concepts are open-textured. Philosophers cannot answer the moral questions concerned with birth and respect for human life, but they can help to show more clearly what the questions involve and that they require human invention, not divination.

Aristotle held that for the solution of practical problems one needs a good character guided by practical intelligence, or wisdom. Wisdom requires knowledge, experience, sound judgement, clear deliberation; there is no short cut. Issues are complex, relevant factors many and varying from case to case, so that no ready-made solutions are available. 'Judgement is in perception', said Aristotle, by which he meant that only when faced with a concrete situation could one make a sound decision, though he did not mean that general principles were irrelevant. Here he is surely right.

So, I think, the medical profession will have to invent its own moral guidelines with regard to the many problems arising from the unparalleled developments in medicine in recent times. Such guidelines will be invented, come what may. If they are to be good guidelines the responsible members of the profession must do what they are no doubt doing, which is to discuss the problems and possible answers in as clear-sighted a way as they can. Only they have the experience and knowledge to judge, and the responsibility will be theirs. If they wish to invite others, including moral philosophers to share in their debates and make what contribution they can, well and good. Certainly no solutions to the issues that cannot command the respect of the community at large will be satisfactory. But they would be stupid to expect to find a solution to their problems given to them as a gift.

But one must be clear that, like all invented laws, rules and regulations, such guidelines cannot be respecters of hard cases. There are times when it might be better to break the law, whatever it may be; it is better to cross double white lines than to run over a child if those are the only options. To think that causing the death of an innocent person or denying the right of a woman to do what she pleases with her body could never be justified is possible only for the enviably inexperienced and unenviably unimaginative. We break wisely made regulations only at our moral, as well as our legal, peril. The dilemma that can here arise is part of the inescapable human predicament.

13   Quality of life and health care

Roger Crisp

Quality-Adjusted-Life-Years

In recent years, Alan Williams and certain other health economists have been developing the notion of a QALY in the hope that it might supply a sound and rational basis for various decisions which medical practitioners and administrators are often required to make.[1] That hope, given the caprice of many such decisions at present, seems to me an admirable one. The foundation of their project is, as far as one can make out, consistently utilitarian. The QALY is offered as a criterion by which the most efficient of various outcomes can, and indeed ought to be, selected.[2] Behind the advocacy of the QALY, then, lies what Philippa Foot has called the compelling and 'rather simple thought that it can never be right to prefer a worse state of affairs to a better'.[3] I myself find this thought compelling.

Before proceeding, I should make clear what I understand by a QALY. Williams himself gives the following account:

[W]e need a simple, versatile, measure of success which incorporates both life expectancy and quality of life, and which reflects the values and ethics of the community served. The ... QALY ... measure fulfils such a role.

The essence of a QALY is that it takes a year of healthy life expectancy to be worth 1, but regards a year of unhealthy life expectancy as worth less than 1. Its precise value is lower the worse the quality of life of the unhealthy person (which is what the 'quality adjusted' bit is all about). If being dead is worth zero, it is, in principle, possible for a QALY to be negative, i.e. for the quality of someone's life to be judged as worse than being dead.

The general idea is that a beneficial health care activity is one that generates a positive amount of QALYs, and an efficient health care activity is one where the cost-per-QALY is as low as it can be.[4]

I shall call the view that we ought to maximize QALYs as so characterized Theory Q. Q can be employed either at the prudential (intrapersonal) level, or at the moral (interpersonal) level. In the former case, for instance, in choosing between two possible operations for myself, I may assess them in terms of the number of QALYs generated by each. In the latter, if I am in charge of a renal dialysis unit with limited resources, I

171

may use Q to decide which patients are to receive treatment. These examples are, of course, only two of many.

The value of health

As I have said, Q can be used as a basis for both prudential and moral decisions. Each of the problems I shall discuss arises at both levels.

The first arises from an over-emphasis on health, at the expense of other values.

Here is a prudential example:

Anna. Anna lives in town T, and requires short but frequent periods of hospitalization if she is to remain in full health. T does not have the facilities to help her. But if she moves to town U, she will be able to obtain suitable care. And her mental health would be unaffected by a move. Anna is engaged in an important and long-term municipal project in town T, where she is heavily involved with the local community. But if she remains there, she will suffer a small drop in her level of health.

Even if we assume that Anna's condition has no effect on her life-expectancy, a doctor advising her on the basis of Q must suggest that, for her own good, she move. Given that he has been asked for prudential advice (advice taking only her own interests into account), the doctor is right not to take into account the effect on the community of Anna's departure. But he is surely wrong to advise her to leave in her own interests. For if she goes, she will lose something deeply important to her – her part in a project to which she may already have dedicated many years, and her relationships with fellow members of the community.

Here is my first moral example of the over-emphasis on health:

The Government Minister. The Chancellor of the Exchequer is deciding on allocations of tax-revenue. She is considering the appropriate levels of funding for the Health Service, education, and the arts.

On the basis of Q, regardless of the general health of the population, all, or most, of the money is likely to be spent on the Health Service. For education and the arts do not have a great effect on our health.

The Q-Theorist may argue that her theory is not intended for decisions at such a high level. I can see no justification for restricting the scope of Q in this way. But even if we allow Q to be confined to the allocation of resources *within* the Health Service, problems will arise. Consider this case:

Baby Brian and Catherine. A doctor at a hospital has a decision to make. Her resources are limited, and she can operate either on Brian, extending his life by two years, or on Catherine, extending hers by one. Brian is one year old. Catherine is middle-aged. Like Anna, Catherine is involved in an important long-term project, which is nearing completion.

The verdict of Q is clear: Brian is to be saved. But this strikes me as quite mistaken. If Catherine is allowed another year, she will be able not only to see the fruits of her labours, but also to tie up any unfinished emotional business in her life. If she dies, her life will end like a bridge which reaches only half-way across a river. The tragedy of Brian's death is different. Whether he dies now or in two years, he will not have been given the chance even of beginning to build bridges.

How can the Q-Theorist avoid problems like these? It must be by putting health into its proper evaluative perspective, along with other things which increase the quality of people's lives, such as their relationships with others, what they accomplish, education and so on. A richer account of what quality of life consists in is required.[5] This richer account can be incorporated into Q, leaving its other principles intact. I shall call the version of Q which is gradually revised throughout this chapter Theory Q*.

The nature of quality

Q is a theory developed in the sphere of welfare economics. It is not surprising, therefore, to find that two of the assumptions on which Q rests are:

... that it is possible to elicit meaningful valuation statements from people about differing degrees of ill-health ... [and] to aggregate these individual valuations in a manner which is consistent with the ethical and political bases of the health-care system.[6]

In the prudential sphere, we are to take the patient's quality of life to be maximized if she gets what she most desires. And at the moral level (particularly in questions of macro-allocation), we are to take into account 'community-evaluations'.[7]

This view about what constitutes quality of life is a subjective one. (Presumably, if spelled out, it would be that a person's life goes better for her the higher the level of the fulfilment of her actual desires, weighted for strength, during her life as a whole. I shall call this the Actual Desire Theory. This theory is open to objection in two places: first, in its focus upon *actual* desire, and, second, in its focus on *desire* itself.

Any theory which rests on the claim that quality of life consists in the fulfilment of desires must have as an implication that the desires fulfilled are actual (existent) desires, *when they are fulfilled*. The 'actual' of the

Actual Desire Theory, then, is not to be seen as opposed to, say, 'hypothetical'.

What, then, is intended by 'actual' desires? Actual desires are desires taken as they are, uncorrected by rationality. The assumption on which the Actual Desire Theory is based is that a person is, by definition, the best judge of what is in her own best interests. Here, what she believes to be so is so.

Very often, however, people are ignorant of straightforward facts. I may desire to spend my summer holiday in Bognor. But if you were to fulfil my desire, it would not make me better off. For I mistakenly think that Bognor is in Tunisia, where I might enjoy the sun.

The Q-Theorist is likely to say here that a person must be supplied with the relevant information if we are to elicit from her the right answer concerning what will most increase the quality of her life. Thus, in a prudential medical case, we should first inform the patient of the likely consequences of her choosing particular courses of action, and make her familiar with such conceptual tools as the Rosser and Kind scales of disability and distress.[8]

But we have now moved away from the Actual Desire Theory to a form of Corrected Desire Theory, in which what a person believes will increase her quality of life cannot be assumed to do so unless she is in possession of relevant information. Following a recent exponent of such a view – James Griffin – let us call a theory, which states that the subject must be fully informed, an Informed Desire Theory.[9] The constraints Griffin puts on desires being informed are very strict:

[A]n 'informed' desire is one formed by appreciation of the nature of its object, and it includes anything necessary to achieve it.[10]

Now recall what I said above about Desire Theories. Such theories require that if something is to add to the quality of my life, it must fulfil a desire that I have. So if I can find a case where a person's quality of life is increased by something which does not fulfil a desire, I will have shown any Desire Theory to be inadequate. I believe the following to be such a case:

The Two Artists. Debbie and Ella are artists. Neither particularly enjoys painting. They practise their art merely to make a living, and both succeed in this to the same degree. Debbie's paintings are inspired and profound, while Ella's are fashionable kitsch.[11]

It is important to remember that it is not relevant to the purpose of this example whether other people see the paintings or not. Imagine first that no one in fact appreciates the paintings, either during or after Debbie's life (the buyers are pure investors). It still seems to me that she has increased the quality of her life through the sheer creation of these works. It is a cheapening of the value of artistic creation to cash it out entirely in terms of the effect that it has on others. If Shakespeare's works had fallen into obscurity, would his accomplishment have had no value *for him*? And if it would have had value, would that value be fully explained by the fact that he fulfilled a desire to write great plays?

Consider next the case where others do appreciate Debbie's works. Here it is even more difficult to deny that Debbie has accomplished something great with her life. She is a painter known to be of the first rate, who gives much pleasure to others. Not only, however, could she not care less about the quality of her work, but she lacks vanity to such an extent that she feels the same way about the opinions of others. In addition, she is selfish enough to be neutral about whether or not her work gives pleasure to others.

Unusual as this example might be, I think that it shows that there is more to quality of life than desire-fulfilment. It demonstrates that there are objective values, which, if instantiated in a person's life, will increase the quality of that life. A plausible theory of quality of life will not emphasize desire, but comprise a list of objective values. I shall call such a theory, after Derek Parfit, an Objective List Theory.[12]

There is a further problem with the Informed Desire Theory, which again points the way to an Objective List Theory. The assumption underlying the Informed Desire Theory is that, with the correct information in front of me, I cannot help but desire what will most increase the quality of my life (for what I most desire *is* that which will most increase quality).

But there are cases where this assumption appears mistaken. One sort of case is mentioned by Parfit in this connection. These are bizarre examples, such as the Rawlsian mathematician whose informed desire is to spend his life counting blades of grass.[13] The difficulty with employing such examples against Informed Desire Theorists is that they look so implausible. And if we accept that a person might make such a choice under conditions of full information, we would surely be inclined to say that she was in some way neurotic. But if we choose more plausible examples – a person, say, who elects to spend her life collecting stamps instead of becoming a successful politician – then the case against the Informed Desire Theory looks weaker. For it might well be that the life of stamp-collecting is the best life for such a person, and that it is only my prejudice which causes me to think otherwise.

But why should we accept desire, even of the informed variety, as the final arbiter of a person's quality of life? For, surely, people do make mistakes in their evaluations, even when they are fully aware of the relevant non-evaluative facts. For example, in certain cases of weakness of will, a person will say: 'I know that option *a* will increase the quality of my life more than option *b*, but it is *b* that I desire more'. Desires do not answer to the facts in a manner reliable enough to qualify them as final arbiters of quality of life. We see this often enough in our own lives. I have a strong desire for the cream cake on the table in front of me. But then I reflect upon the situation. I have high blood-pressure, and my doctor has told me to avoid foods with a high fat content. Has my desire diminished in the light of my reflection? Not – in this case – in the slightest. Irrationality, in the sense of a lack of responsiveness to beliefs, seems built into the conative side of human nature.

It might be said that, in cases like this, the desire on which decisions are based is uninformed.

There is a question here about the nature of the information required for rational assessment of quality of life. The Informed Desire Theorist can be confronted with a dilemma.

If we take her claims at face value, and interpret her as stipulating that the information be non-evaluative, she will be impaled on the first horn. For, even if the blade-counter case is of doubtful import, it is hard to deny that people do make mistakes, and that desire does not respond fully to the facts.

If the Informed Desire Theorist were to specify, however, that the information can be partly evaluative in nature, such as that *x is better than y*, she would be impaled on the second horn. And at two points.

First, although she could now deal with cases of mistaken judgement (the stamp-collector does not know that the political life is in her best interests), a solution to the problem raised by the type of weakness of will I have outlined will elude her still. For such weak-willed people know which is the better course of action. And yet their desire is for the less valuable alternative.

Second, and more seriously, this account is a Desire Theory in name only. For if the desires of the blade-counter, the stamp-collector, and the cake-lover are described as uninformed, it seems to make the criterion for a desire's being informed something like its being a desire shaped by a recognition of what is quite *independent* of desire. Such a theory is too objective to count as a Desire Theory. It is a form of Objective List.

But how is all this abstract argument relevant to Q, which is a theory designed to aid those involved in practical decision-making? Again, it does not amount to an objection to *any* theory on the lines of Q. What I have argued is that the Q-Theorist's conception of quality of life is too subjective. But Q* can incorporate an Objective List. And this would have practical consequences.

At the prudential level, we should of course endeavour to supply to any particular patient as much relevant information and time for reflection upon it as we can. But the rôle of the doctor should not consist just in this. She should not function as a market-researcher, but as a counsellor, seeing herself and the patient as engaged in the joint project of discovering what is best for the latter. There is a need for persons skilled both in medical practice, and in the analytical skills of moral philosophy. Medicine and moral reasoning should go hand in hand.[14]

At the moral level, we must avoid the sin of many objective theories – the violation of autonomy. I have not discussed the content of any particular Objective List, but it seems to me that any theory which does not count autonomy as an important value will be out of the running. But neither should we take decisions concerning the allocation of medical resources purely on the basis of revealed preferences. For preferences can be irrational. For example, I (and many others) might want operation x in preference to operation y because a famous pop star made that choice. What people want is only one factor in these questions, albeit the most important. Administrators, too, must consider the real effects of their decisions on the quality of people's lives. And because their rôle should be more active, they must be open and answerable to us. Such decisions are best made in the context of a stable democracy. Here, then, is a further place where politics influences health care.

Repugnant conclusions

Even a version of Q which is based on a richer and more objective account of the QALY will run into further trouble. It leads to conclusions of the kind that Parfit has called 'repugnant'.[15] We can describe Repugnant Conclusions either as Theoretical or as Practical. Theoretical Repugnant Conclusions are those to which a theory is committed, yet the situations envisaged in which are highly unlikely to occur. Such conclusions are still problematic for the theories which lead to them. A Practical Repugnant Conclusion concerns possibilities which it is quite conceivable may become actual in the world. I shall give four Repugnant Conclusions of Q.

Theoretical Prudential Repugnant Conclusion. For any possible lifetime of eighty years at a very high quality of life, there must be some much longer life, the quality of which is such as to make it barely worth living, and yet which, other things being equal, would be better.

Theoretical Moral Repugnant Conclusion. For any possible population of at least ten billion people, all with a very high quality of life, there must be some

much larger imaginable population whose existence, if other things are equal, would be better, even though its members have lives that are barely worth living.[16]
Practical Prudential Repugnant Conclusion. Sixty years of life of a very low quality (0.2) are better than fifteen years of a very high quality (0.75).
Practical Moral Repugnant Conclusion. If we are faced with two alternative policies:
(a) saving, for one extra year each, one hundred people who are going to die without treatment in five years;
(b) saving two people for forty-five years,
we should choose (a).

Once again, the fact that Q implies these conclusions need not spell its utter demise. For if we introduce three connected notions into our analysis of quality of life, Q* can avoid Repugnant Conclusions. These notions have been plausibly developed by Griffin.[17] The first is:

The Global Conception. We can never reach final assessment of ways of life by totting up lots of small, short-term utilities.[18]

When we are assessing the quality of a life, we have to step back and reflect upon the life as a whole. For example, we may judge that sixty years at level 0.2 is *not* better than fifteen at 0.75.

The Q-Theorist will, of course, now accuse me of straightforward mathematical error ($60 \times 0.2 = 12$; $15 \times 0.75 = 11.25$). Let me introduce the second notion I have in mind:

The Formal Conception. 'Utility' ... is not to be seen as the single over-arching value, in fact not as a substantive value at all, but instead as a formal analysis of what it is for something to be prudentially valuable to some person.[19]

What constitutes the quality of life, then, is not a substantive super-value like pleasure. Quality is not like milk. Milk is a substance, so that if one has two bottles containing 1 litre each, one has the same amount of milk as someone with 2,000 bottles containing 1 ml. each.

Quality consists in the values on the Objective List being instantiated in a person's life. And these values, although irreducibly plural, are not incommensurable in any strong sense. Trade-offs are not impossible. I may decide to sacrifice some of my autonomy in order to deepen a personal relationship. But I do not make my decision by means of weighing up some substratum common to both. 'Judgement lies in one's perception.'[20]

When we take into account the Global and Formal Conceptions of quality, and the fact that we find the conclusions above so repugnant, we are able to see that there is a third notion in play:

Discontinuity. There are ... incommensurabilities of the form: enough of A outweighs any amount of B.[21]

If I were offered a full human lifetime of eighty years of life at a high quality, *no* number of years at a far lower quality of life could ever constitute a more valuable option for me. I should judge the first lifetime better, even if the second were eternal. This insight occurs when I take the evaluative step back (the Global Conception), and realize that value is not some substantive, dominant end (the Formal Conception).

Thus, if Q* is based on the Global and Formal Conceptions of quality, and the view that values are discontinuous, it can avoid Repugnant Conclusions both in theory and in practice.

Fairness

But there still remains a final problem for Q-Theories. According to Q and Q*, the *objectively* right thing to do is to maximize QALYs.[22] Imagine that I am a doctor who specializes in an unusual and highly risky form of surgery. I am introduced to a patient who, if operated upon by me, will have another fifty years of life of a high quality (at level 1). But, on the basis of sound statistical evidence, it is clear that there is a chance of only about one in a hundred that the operation will succeed. If it fails, my patient will die. And if not operated upon, it is almost certain that she will live for ten years at level 1, and then die. If I operate, and the operation is successful, according to Q and Q* I have performed the objectively right action. For I have produced the highest possible number of QALYs.

But, of course, I did not know that the operation would succeed. It was pure luck. And if I tried the same trick one hundred times, the chances are that ninety-nine people would die. We are in fact required to aim to perform the *subjectively* best action. To do this involves taking probabilities into account. We are to maximize the *expected* number of QALYs. The process of calculation involves taking the number of QALYs which will be produced by a certain outcome, and multiplying that number by the probability of its occurrence. In the above case, I should have reasoned as follows:

Operate: $0.01 \times 50 = 0.5$
Not operate: $1 \times 10 = 10$

Even taking the figures as approximate, it is clear that I should have refrained from operating in this instance.

The final problem for Q* arises when we combine the notion of maximizing *expected* QALYs with that of discontinuity. It seems that the theory is faced with further undesirable or unacceptable conclusions. Consider this prudential case:

The Undesirable Conclusion. It would be unwise for me to take a leisurely drive into the country on Sunday afternoon.

The reasoning behind this is as follows. I judge that *no* amount of the pleasure to be gained from such recreation could be more valuable than the remainder of my life. As a rational QALY-maximizer in my own life, I must take into account the admittedly very small probability of my being killed in a car-crash. Let us say that the chance is one in a million. Given that I must attempt to maximize QALYs, my reasoning must be as follows:

$$q \times 0.999999 < r \times 0.000001,$$

where q is the quality added to my life by the drive, and r the value of my lifetime as a whole. What is remarkable here is that the form of the equation will remain the same until the number on the right-hand side reaches zero. In other words, even if the chance of my death is one in ten billion, I should still remain at home. This is because of the discontinuity between q and r. r is more valuable than infinitely many qs. Discontinuities in value introduce the irrationality of infinitesimal mathematics into maximizing theories.

But here the Q*-Theorist may bring our attention once again to the Global and Formal Conceptions. If we adopt these, we are enabled to avoid the Undesirable Conclusion. For if I step back, I can see that a life in which I engage in such pursuits as driving for pleasure now and again, even taking into account the risks, is far more valuable than a life in which I spend my time cooped up in a room trying to avoid death. We should not maximize occasion-by-occasion in the way suggested by the Undesirable Conclusion.

Let us accept this reply, for the sake of argument, and move from the prudential to the moral sphere. Here we seem to be faced with Unacceptable Conclusions:

The First Unacceptable Conclusion. If I am a member of the Cave Rescue Organization, and I know of a person paralyzed and seriously brain-damaged at the bottom of a cave well-known to me, I should not attempt a rescue.

The reasoning here is analogous to that underlying the Undesirable Conclusion. Let us assume that I have only a one in a million chance of death. Then,

$$s \times 0.999999 < t \times 0.000001,$$

where s is the value of the life of the paralyzed person, and t the value of my own life. Because of the discontinuity in value between my life and that of the injured person – no number of seriously brain-damaged lives could counterbalance the value of my own lifetime – I ought not to risk my life for the injured caver.

The following illustrates a medical implication of Q*:

The Second Unacceptable Conclusion. Other things being equal (*i.e.* there being no bad side-effects), we should remove all but very basic funding from support for the severely mentally defective, and use it to decrease risks of death for non-defective people.

Again, as long as the probability numbers on the right-hand side of the equation are above zero, the conclusion follows. Therefore, however great the loss in quality of life of severely mentally defective people, and however little the risk of death avoided, we should channel funding away from the severely mentally defective. Let us assume that there is a one in a hundred million chance that a person will be killed by an adder each year. Then however devastating the consequences might be, Q* implies that we should use resources now employed to help the severely mentally defective for adder-extermination. For, faced in imagination with the choice of living the lives in question in random serial order, I will point to the lost life in the UK every two years and judge that *no* number of severely mentally defective lives at whatever level would counterbalance the value of that non-defective lifetime.[23]

This time, in the moral sphere, the Q*-Theorist cannot urge me to adopt the Global Conception in assessing the value of the lives in question. For I am already doing so. I am considering the life of the adder-victim *and* the lives of the mentally-defective persons in a global manner.

What seems to be happening is that I am totting up at the moral level the value of lives assessed globally at the prudential level. To avoid the Unacceptable Conclusions, it appears that we must adopt a certain *Meta-global* outlook at the moral level. Here, Q* runs into its final, and, as far as I can see, insurmountable, problem. It cannot offer us an outlook which avoids Unacceptable Conclusions. For such conclusions rest on Q*'s Meta-global outlook – that we should maximize QALYs. To avoid those conclusions, the Meta-global outlook has to differ structurally from a mere extension of the Totting-up Conception into the moral sphere. Moral positions based on fairness, perhaps, can offer a more plausible Meta-global outlook than that of Q*.[24] At the moral level, seeing things Meta-globally, a society in which mentally defective people receive substantial support appears fairer than one in which they are ignored for the sake of eliminating small risks of death for non-defective people.

If the above argument is correct, the maximizing assumptions on which Q* is based make that theory morally unacceptable as it stands. Account should be taken of considerations of fairness.[25]

Conclusion

I have argued that a theory which requires us to maximize QALYs should (1) put health into its evaluative perspective; (2) be based on an Objective List of values; (3) incorporate the Global and Formal Conceptions of quality, as well as the notion of Discontinuity; (4) make room for considerations of fairness.

ACKNOWLEDGEMENTS

I am grateful to David Edmonds, James Griffin, Martha Klein and Michael Lockwood for helpful comments on earlier drafts.

NOTES

1 See e.g. A. Williams (1985) 'The value of QALYs', *Health and Social Service Journal*, 18 July; 'Economics of coronary artery bypass grafting', *British Medical Journal* 291, pp. 326–9.

2 When I speak of a 'QALY', I mean either a QALY or the notion of a QALY. The context should make clear the meaning in each case.

3 P. Foot (1985) 'Utilitarianism and the virtues', *Mind* 94, p. 198. See A. Williams (1984) 'Health service efficiency and clinical freedom', *Nuffield/York Portfolio*, p. 8: '... our guiding principle is the entirely "ethical" one of ensuring that the benefits gained outweigh the benefits forgone'.

4 Williams (1985) 'The value of QALYs', p. 3.

5 I should point out here that Williams himself countenances the possibility of an age-adjusted QALY. See 'Welfare economics and health status measurement' in J. van der Gaag and M. Perlman (eds.) (1981) *Health, Economics, and Health Economics*, Amsterdam: North-Holland Publishing Co., p. 276; and 'The value of QALYs', p. 5. But on p. 4 of the latter, he rules out consideration of 'higher things'. *Anna* and *The Government Minister* would therefore still constitute problems for his view.

6 Williams (1985) 'The value of QALYs', *Health and Social Service Journal*, 18 July, p. 4.

7 Williams (1981) 'Welfare economics and health status measurement', p. 276; Williams (1984) 'Health service efficiency and clinical freedom', p. 3.

8 R. Rosser and P. Kind (1978) 'A scale of valuations of states of illness: is there a social consensus?', *International Journal of Epidemiology* 7, 1978.

9 J. Griffin (1986) *Well-Being*. Oxford: Clarendon Press, pp. 11–15.

10 *Ibid.*, p. 14.

11 I have discussed this case and its implications further in Crisp (1990) 'Sidgwick and self-interest', *Utilitas* 2, pp. 274–6.

12 D. Parfit (1984) *Reasons and Persons*. Oxford: Clarendon Press, p. 493.

13 *Ibid.*, pp. 499–500; see J. Rawls (1972) *A Theory of Justice*. Oxford: Oxford University Press, p. 432.

14 I have argued the case for the introduction of a new medical specialization –

telostrics – combining clinical, philosophical and social work rôles in the care of the dying in *Bioethics* 1, 1987.

15 Parfit (1984) *Reasons and Persons*, pp. 381–90. The term 'repugnant' is used in connection with such a conclusion in J. McTaggart (1927) *The Nature of Existence*, Cambridge University Press, vol. II, pp. 452–3. McTaggart himself does not find such conclusions repugnant.

16 Quoted from Parfit (1984) *Reasons and Persons*. Oxford: Clarendon Press, p. 388.

17 The following is necessarily abridged and unclear. I can only recommend the reader to consult Griffin (1986) *Well-Being*. Oxford: Clarendon Press. See especially ch. 2, §5; ch. 9, §3 (on the Global Conception); ch. 2, §4 (on the Formal Conception); ch. 5, §6; ch. 11, §9 (on Discontinuity). On the latter notion, see also H. Rashdall (1907) *The Theory of Good and Evil*, Oxford: Clarendon Press, vol. II, pp. 38–41. The relation between the Repugnant Conclusion and Discontinuity is explored in Griffin (1986) *Well-Being*, note 27, p. 338; and Parfit (1986) 'Overpopulation and the quality of life' in P. Singer (ed.) *Applied Ethics*. Oxford: Oxford University Press.

18 Griffin (1986) *Well-Being*. Oxford: Clarendon Press, p. 34.

19 *Ibid.*, pp. 31–2.

20 R. Crisp (1994) Aristotle, *Ethica Nicomachea*. Oxford: Clarendon Press, Book II, ch. 9, 1109b23.

21 Griffin (1986) *Well-Being*. Oxford: Clarendon Press, p. 89.

22 On the 'objective/subjective' distinction here, see H. Sidgwick (1907) *The Methods of Ethics*. London: Macmillan, 7th edn, pp. 207–8.

23 The notion of comparing in imagination lives lived in random serial order as a method of interpersonal comparison is taken from C. I. Lewis (1946) *An Analysis of Knowledge and Valuation*. La Salle, IL: Open Court, pp. 546–7.

24 I use the term 'fairness' for lack of a better alternative. Admittedly, like much of what I say in this paragraph, the notion of fairness is vague. I am leaving a great deal of unfinished business. My aim, however, is to show that there is work to be done.

25 Considerations of justice and fairness in relation to the QALY are discussed in J. Harris (1987) 'QALYfying the value of life', *Journal of Medical Ethics* 13; and M. Lockwood (1988) 'Quality of life and resource allocation', in J. M. Bell and S. Mendus (eds.) *Philosophy and Medical Welfare*. Cambridge: Cambridge University Press.

14   Dependency: the foundational value in medical ethics

Alastair V. Campbell

In this chapter I am seeking to correct a rank order of moral principles which seems to have crept into the literature of medical ethics over the past two decades, almost unobserved. There has developed a presumption in favour of individual self-determination or autonomy, and an implied or explicit criticism of the beneficent approach to the health care relationship as being second best, or justified only in certain strictly demarcated circumstances. Examples of this ordering of principles are not hard to find in the standard works in contemporary medical ethics.[1] A notable counterbalancing of this prevailing view-point has been Pellegrino and Thomasma's *For the Patient's Good: The Restoration of Beneficence in Health Care*.[2] To some extent this chapter can be seen as an elaboration of some aspects of their argument. But my central point is perhaps more controversial than theirs. I want to assert that the fundamental character of human life is one of dependency, and that therefore a medical ethics which seeks to overemphasise the independence of the individual is in danger of being a de-humanising and inadequate account of the therapeutic relationship. I have already stated this fundamental assumption about the dependent nature of human existence in my book, *Moderated Love*. Writing about the 'wisdom' upon which medical interventions must be based, I described the following features of the 'creatureliness' which constitutes human life:

> To be a creature is to be born of others, to know ourselves through them, to depend upon them and create dependency, to know the pain of losing them and finally to be the instance of that pain to others.[3]

This description may at first appear to depend upon theological rather than ethical assumptions, since the concept of 'creatureliness' implies a creator upon whom life itself is dependent. But although it is true that I would add this extra dimension of dependency on God to my account of human nature, it is not essential to an ethical argument promoting the pre-eminence of dependency in human life. My statement firstly describes an empirical state. Humans *are* dependent on other humans throughout most

184

or all of their lives. In describing this as 'creatureliness' I accept that I am also making an evaluative claim. I am claiming that such dependency is a good state, one which fulfils and enhances our God-given humaneness. In this chapter, however, I shall try to establish that claim without resort to the theological statements. I shall argue that there are good arguments of a personalist kind to put this aspect of human life in the forefront of our shared human experience. This will lead me to put a higher value on beneficence than it currently receives in arguments about how medicine is rightly practised. My perspective on the moral context of medical care is close to that of Stanley Hauerwas, as expressed in his collection of essays, *Suffering Presence*:

Medicine involves the needs and interests that we all share. All of us wish to avoid untimely death. All wish to avoid unnecessary suffering. All wish to be cared for when we are hurt . . . Medicine provides a powerful reminder . . . of our 'nature' as bodily beings beset by illness and destined for death. Yet medicine also reminds us it is our 'nature' to be a community that refuses to let suffering alienate us from one another. The crucial question is what kind of community we should be to be capable of that task.[4]

The answer to Hauerwas' question, as I understand it, is to be a community which can meet the dependency needs of its members at all stages of their development. It is on the bedrock of this community support that individual self-determination is built, and such self-determination is always circumscribed by our fragility and our mortality.

Dependency as a moral good

What then are we to say, in a positive moral sense, of dependency? Let us define it as 'being in relationship to others in a manner which makes them necessary for the fulfilment of some or all of our needs'. The newborn infant provides an example of such dependency: without warmth and nourishment provided by others the child will quickly die. Moreover, psychological study of young babies has demonstrated that the absence of a consistent parenting figure (maternal deprivation) can lead to severe depression which can be literally fatal. Many examples of dependency in adult life can be taken from medical practice, ranging from the dependency created by trauma, to the deliberately induced dependency of anaesthesia prior to surgery. In these examples there is really little to discuss: the dependency is necessary and inevitable, and, in order to maintain the life and promote the health of the individual, dependency must be acknowledged and the needs met. But it can be argued that all illness creates at least a period of necessary dependency. This is well described by Oliver Sacks in *A Leg to Stand On*:

> though as a sick patient, in hospital, one was reduced to moral infancy, this was not a malicious degradation, but a biological and spiritual need of the hurt creature. One had to go back, one had to regress, for one might indeed be as helpless as a child, whether one liked it, or willed it, or not. In hospital one became again a child with parents (parents who might be good or bad), and this might be felt as 'infantilising' and degrading, or as a sweet and sorely needed nourishing.[5]

So far I have been describing examples of unsought dependency. But it is where the possibility of choice enters in or appears to enter in that we become less sure of the place of dependency in the moral scheme of things. Should we *create* dependency upon ourselves? Should we *seek to be* dependent on others? Or should we shun dependency whenever we are capable of doing so, regarding the beneficent relationship in health care as always demeaning and 'paternalistic'?

Much of the confusion about these issues stems from the tendency of the medical ethics literature to focus on the dramatic situations of critical care medicine. These, of course, do present the individual with massive threats to his or her independence and provoke major questions about the extent to which professional power can be abused in numerous ways when the patient is helpless in bed or on the operating table. But the most dramatic is not necessarily a good representation of the most common experience of illness or disability in everyday human life. Much experience of illness is less well-defined, has less clear ending and finishing points, and creates relationships with others of an important but less potentially threatening kind. Thus, for virtually everyone, the most common illness experiences will be such things as the common cold, headaches of ill-defined origin, muscular pains, general feelings of low mood or depression. The high drama of modern hospital medicine has virtually nothing to contribute to an understanding of the appropriate care of individuals in these common experiences of ill-health. Yet such experiences are the ones which we must learn to incorporate in our everyday lives to an increasing degree as we progress from youth to age. We need to learn how to cope with a series of minor ailments in ourselves and in those on whom we depend (or who depend on us). To illustrate this point further I shall consider two examples in which the dependency of everyday life is inevitably increased by the presence of chronic illness or disability. By moving from these examples (rather than from critical care examples) we may see more clearly the moral character of the dependent relationship.

The dependent relative

The phenomenon of the dependent relative is not one which is discussed much in medical ethics – reflecting no doubt its hospital-biassed and crisis-based origins. Yet here is an area where the community concern for the vulnerable is really put to the test. As the age profile of the populations of industrialised nations shifts to an ever-increasing elderly group, the phenomenon of dependency in *adult* life cannot be overlooked. Despite a popular impression to the contrary only a tiny proportion of the over-65 age group in the UK is in institutional care. (1.6 per cent are in residential care permanently: 2.1 per cent of them are permanently in hospital, about 5 per cent are either in hospital or residential care, temporarily or permanently, at any one time.) Of course, a very large proportion of the remaining 95 per cent of the over-65s are not in need of special care, but it is clear that there are very significant numbers of people who do require care and who are not in any kind of institutional setting.

Who then are the principal carers of this dependent non-institutionalised elderly group? An Equal Opportunities Survey published in 1982 found that 42 per cent of them were themselves over 60 (72 per cent over 50) and that the vast majority were women. Moreover, the lower the socioeconomic class, the more severe the dependency was likely to be and the less likely it was that the carer would have good access to support services.

What conclusions might we draw from this example? Firstly, it illustrates that the phenomenon of permanent dependency is much more widespread than the 'blood and glory' style of medical ethics may chose to notice, and that this is likely to increase in the foreseeable future, thanks to the 'success' of life-saving or life-prolonging medicine. Of course dependency in this context is (or should be) only a part of the whole picture. An ethic which stresses respect for the wishes of the elderly, enhancement of their capabilities and the encouragement of independence is undoubtedly of central importance (and needs constant imaginative revitalisation.) But none of this can take away from the obvious vulnerability of the old and their need for a network of supporters, both professional and non-professional. Secondly, the vulnerability of the principal carers (relatives who are themselves advanced in years) needs to be taken note of. Who cares for the carers? In a society where independence is regarded as supremely to be valued, those who seem to be coping are seen as moral exemplars – and left to get on with it. Thirdly, the inequality of the burden of care should be noted. Ill-health is much more prevalent in the social class where the obligation to sacrifice oneself to care for a relative is likely to be more strongly felt and where the economic resources to enlist other help do not exist. The extremes of this inequality are the outcome of a political philosophy of *laissez-faire* liberalism, and it is this philosophy which has encouraged the predominance of individual autonomy as a guiding moral principle.

The intellectually handicapped

My second example entails a still more radical critique of the kind of society which stresses competence and self-sufficiency. It comes from the later sections of Hauerwas' *Suffering Presence*, in which he attacks current trends towards the elimination of intellectual handicap from society through selective abortion or new techniques in reproductive medicine. Hauerwas believes that the argument that thereby we are preventing suffering is a spurious one (for we imagine that to be intellectually handicapped is to be ourselves with normal faculties in that state of dependency). Instead, he argues, our real reason for wanting to eliminate intellectual handicap is that we do not wish to face the moral challenge which it represents. We cherish our own self-possession and independence. But our basic state is in reality a very vulnerable one. We need others to ensure our own survival and identity. Because we are loath to admit this neediness, we 'disdain those who do not or cannot cover up their neediness. Prophetlike, the retarded only remind us of the insecurity hidden in our false sense of self-possession.'[6]

Hauerwas' argument is in danger of being a serious over-simplification of the issues. Most obviously, he fails to make plain what degree of intellectual handicap he has in mind. He could be guilty of the idealisation of some truly miserable states in reaction to an increasingly eugenic approach to the society of the future. But without undue sentimentalising, there is still much to be learned from the intellectually handicapped. Do we genuinely respect and wish to learn from those whose autonomy is so severely restricted that they depend upon consistent daily stimulation to achieve any source of independence and choice? Obviously we will find the rational and self-regulating person easier to deal with than people of impaired intelligence and poor impulse control. Perhaps, too, we feel threatened by the total commitment and trustworthiness which such vulnerable beings demand of us. But the experience of relating to the intellectually handicapped can remind us of the arrogance of our self-sufficiency; and the need for focused and individualised concern reminds us of the essential blend of reason and emotion which genuine respect for others entails.

Dependency and autonomy

How then are we to understand the relationship between respect for autonomy (which I do not contest as an important moral principle) and respect for dependency (which, I am arguing, is a more fundamental principle)? We would be mistaken to suppose that dependency and autonomy are polar opposites. A person may be dependent on another yet still exercise autonomy (e.g. as a partner in a marriage in which neither partner seeks to dominate but supports the other). Conversely, a very independent individual could be lacking in autonomy, in the sense that he or she cannot consistently exercise any degree of self-direction and cannot function as a member of society. As Kant perceived, autonomy entails the capacity to live in an interactive community of moral agents. Thus the converse of autonomy is not dependency, but heteronomy, a state in which the individual has lost or abandoned the capacity for self-determination.

The essential characteristics of autonomy are well summarised by Harris:

critical self-determination in which the agent strives to make decisions which are as little marred by defects in reason, information or control as she can make them.[7]

The abandonment of autonomy is thus more than simply 'rule by another'. It is the loss of that decision-making capacity which makes us moral agents. This point is well made by Richard Lindley. Observing that heteronomy, like (say) baldness, is rarely an absolute state, but more a matter of degree, Lindley suggests that we judge a person's degree of autonomy/heteronomy on both cognitive and conative criteria. A person is *cognitively* heteronomous, either if she holds a set of beliefs which are false, or if the beliefs are held without the active exercise of theoretical reason to establish their truthfulness. A person is *conatively* heteronomous if her actions are determined by desires which she regards as of lesser importance or if she fails to act on what she believes to be her preferred choices ('weakness of the will').[8]

Let it be granted that the features described by Harris and by Lindley are essential components of the moral life. Those aspects of life in community which require of us responsible decision-making are certainly dependent upon the extent to which we are willing or able to exercise autonomous choice and to resist defects of will and of reasoning. The question still remains: are these our first and fundamental obligations as members of the human community? The point is at least contestable. Why should autonomy hold a supreme position in moral theory? Two different kinds of justification have been offered. In Kant's analysis of the 'good will', only the autonomous agent can be said to act in a genuinely moral manner. Thus (as Kant sees it) autonomy must logically hold the pre-eminent position in morality. A different kind of argument is found in the modified utilitarianism of J. S. Mill. According to Mill, a society which does not give priority to individual liberty cannot be one which safeguards the common good. Thus the supreme good is found in the aggregate of autonomous individuals.

Both types of justification depend upon our accepting the prior assumption that morality begins with the individual and his or her personal liberty, and both theories (despite their massive differences in approach), attempt to build a communal morality out of each individual's respect for this freedom. But suppose we were to begin the discussion of the pre-eminence of moral values at a different place – at our interdependence rather than our capacity (or lack of it) for independent choice and action? With such a starting point the predominant obligation would be a respect for the dependency which specific others have upon us, and an attention to the duties which fall upon us as a result of this dependency. Equally we would pay attention to and respect our own dependency upon significant others and seek the support which we knew we required for our own security and fulfilment. With such a starting point, the society most productive of human good would be the one in which the needs of the vulnerable were given preference over the freedom of the strong to exercise maximum liberty of action.

Implications for medical ethics

How might a redefinition of our starting point affect our understanding of medical ethics? The most obvious effect would be a re-ordering of priorities about the kind of problems considered central to the field. We would look in different places for the normative examples for our accounts of ethical theory. Consider the following case, which from the point of view of an ethic-stressing autonomy in an acute medicine setting can be seen as virtually an insoluble problem.

Marie was a frequent inmate of the medical wards of a large hospital. She had persistent and distressing nausea and diarrhoea, unamenable to relief by medication. She had had a battery of tests to establish some cause of her problems, had been interviewed by a psychiatrist to determine if her symptoms were stress related, and (in view of the absence of any other explanation) was now a likely candidate for exploratory surgery, since cancer of the bowel seemed a real possibility. One other possible explanation remained, however. Her symptoms were consistent with regular and excessive use of purgatives. When this diagnosis was put to her, Marie adamantly denied that she ever took medicine of this sort.

The doctor in charge of her case unconvinced by her denials, decided to have her locker searched while she was out of the ward for (yet more) tests. A large container of powerful purgatives was discovered. When confronted with this discovery, Marie was willing to say only that they *could* be an explanation of her problem, but she was never willing to admit directly that she took the purgatives. She was discharged with advice to avoid her symptoms by avoiding taking the purgatives. The doctors expected to see her again. On the basis of previous experience of such cases, they felt sure that her illness was necessary to her. Sooner or later she would return, complaining of the same symptoms.

An extreme case like this forces us to reconsider the way in which we conceptualise the dilemmas of medical ethics. It could reasonably be said that Marie was in a markedly heteronomous state, since her actions were quite out of line with her expressed intentions, to the extent that she could not even admit to them, when challenged about her behaviour. Her doctors reacted to this state by an action which simply disregarded her rights as an autonomous agent. The surreptitious search of her locker was tantamount to treating her as an incompetent child, whose consent to a 'treatment' measure need not be sought. When the confrontation tactic did not have the desired effect, Marie was then cast off as an incurable who could be forgotten for a while, but never properly helped. She failed to fit the categories of modern medical practice. She was seeking to be treated as a person in need, but her 'choices' did not fit the ideal model of the rational, autonomous and co-operative patient. And yet what we see in Marie's case is only a dramatic example of a very common form of behaviour. The need to gain attention through illness is one with which we are all familiar in our own lives. It is a need related to our dependent selves, which in times of stress may take a predominant role in our lives, to a point where we no longer want the burdens of autonomous choice. We want an excuse to 'have a holiday' from our responsibilities. Illness offers a socially acceptable excuse, one which exempts us from accusations of laziness or irresponsibility. An approach to medical ethics which starts with the assumption that people always *want* to be well is incapable of dealing with a very significant part of health care interactions. It is an approach impoverished by a naive form of rationalism, which refuses to recognise the complexity of human behaviour.

What is required in the place of such an overstress on autonomy is a re-affirmation of the beneficent aspects of health care – those aspects which provide protection, nurture and support to those who need a restoration of their power to cope unaided. Such an approach does not commit us to collude in self-destructive behaviour like Marie's. But it recognises that much of the time the ethical challenge is not to demand autonomous responses from ill people, but to find ways of moving them from an inappropriate and self-perpetuating dependency, to a restorative and releasing one. To do this we require more than simply the tools of rational analysis of possible choices of action. We need a relationship of mutual respect and trust between the providers and recipients of health care, based on a communal value which regards care for the weak and vulnerable as a fundamental ethical imperative.

Thus I hope for a revaluation of dependency. To adapt the famous words of Hobbes: a health care ethic which pays no regard to the basic human need for dependency will, in the increasing monetarism of our times, be 'nasty, brutish and short'. It really takes little time to ensure that people take charge of their own lives, *if they can.* It is having the compassion and commitment to help those who have lost the capacity for self-determination that properly tests our moral seriousness as providers of health care rather than mere contractors of medical interventions.

NOTES

1 See especially T. Engelhardt (1986) *The Foundations of Bioethics.* New York: Oxford University Press, but several other widely used textbooks, e.g. Veatch's (1981) *A Theory of Medical Ethics.* New York: Basic Books and Beauchamp and Childress's (1983) *Principles of Biomedical Ethics.* Oxford University Press, show a less marked but similar tendency.
2 Pellegrino, E. D. and Thomasma, D. C. (1988) *For the Patient's Good.* New York: Oxford University Press, 1988.
3 Campbell, A. V. (1984) *Moderated Love.* London: SPCK, p. 96.
4 Hauerwas, S. (1986) *Suffering Presence.* Edinburgh: T & T Clark, p. 7.
5 Sacks, Oliver (1986) *A Leg to Stand On.* London: Pan Books, p. 128.
6 Hauerwas (1986) *Suffering Presence,* p. 169.
7 Harris, J. (1985) *The Value of Life.* London: Routledge and Kegan Paul, p. 212.
8 Lindley, R. (1986) *Autonomy.* London: Macmillan, ch. 5.

15   Not more medical ethics

K. William M. Fulford

Read in one way the title of this chapter is a plea. *Not* more medical ethics! This plea may have a reactionary voice. Not everyone is an enthusiast for the new growth industry which is medical ethics. Yet it may also have a progressive voice. Even among those who are supportive of medical ethics there is a suspicion that, growth industry or not, at the end of the day it will add rather little to the actual practice of medicine.

In this chapter I want to explore the possible contribution to medical ethics of linguistic or conceptual analysis, in particular as this has been concerned with the distinction between fact and value. Some may consider this a philosophically old-fashioned approach. Others may believe that it is too theoretical to be practically useful. However I hope to show that followed through with sufficient determination it can help to bring medical ethics closer to the contingencies of everyday clinical work.

Conceptual difficulties in medicine

The belief that medical ethics has relatively little practical relevance is a facet of what has become known as the medical model. This model is called 'medical' because it is the model (or picture) of medicine that is adopted more or less consciously by most doctors. It amounts to the idea that medicine is essentially a science, and hence that the problems with which doctors are concerned in their everyday clinical work are, at heart, empirical. It is consistent with this science-based view of medicine that doctors should act ethically. It is acknowledged that medical ethics may induce a greater sensitivity to the ethical aspects of clinical work and research. But this is all somewhat peripheral. At the centre of the proper concerns of medicine, it is felt, there is a range of empirical problems to which the traditional medical sciences – anatomy, physiology, bacteriology and so forth – hold all the answers.

This is clearly an over-simple view of medicine. Most doctors recognise that a number of disciplines are relevant to medicine besides the empirical sciences – economics, law, politics and social administration, for instance.

But it is considered that these are not part of the technical expertise of doctors *as* doctors. What is perhaps not so well recognised, however, is that even at the 'scientific' centre of medicine there is more to clinical decision making than just matters of fact. For the very classification of diseases, and with it medical diagnosis, depends not just on the facts but on the construction that is placed on the facts.

It is through this constructive or conceptual element in diagnosis that ethical theory can be shown to have a central, not just peripheral, place in medicine. Consider involuntary psychiatric treatment, for example. Such treatment is ethically contentious (McGarry and Chodoff, 1981). The standard ethical intuition is that in certain cases – suicidal depression, say – it is right to treat a patient against their express wishes, either in that patient's own interests or for the protection of others. This is a strongly held intuition with deep historical roots and one which is shared by many different cultural traditions. It is not universal, however. There are those, like Szasz (1963) and Foucault (1973), who argue that all involuntary treatment is really just a form of social manipulation or political control. These are extreme views. But in everyday practice many cases are marginal or in other ways problematic. There may be differences of opinion in a given case, between doctor and doctor, or between the doctor and others concerned with the patient – nurses, social workers or relatives. Differences of this kind, furthermore, underline the risks of misuse of involuntary treatment; and intentional abuses, sometimes institutionalised (Bloch, 1981), are far from infrequent.

There is thus a practical need for clarification of the grounds of compulsory treatment. According to the medical model, however, the required clarification is not conceptual but empirical. The expectation is that the difficulties surrounding involuntary treatment will be resolved with appropriate developments in the brain sciences. What is problematic about involuntary treatment, however, is in general not the facts but how the facts are to be interpreted. The patient is known to be, say, both depressed and suicidal. What is at issue is whether in virtue of their sadness and their wish for death they are ill. And this question of interpretation cannot be settled even in principle by tests of brain functioning. For the very significance of such tests depends ultimately on the construction that is placed on the patient's symptoms. It may well be that particular patterns of brain functioning will one day be shown to underlie particular experiences and behaviours. But these patterns of brain functioning will only be causes of *illness*, and hence diagnostically significant, if the experiences and behaviours themselves are first construed as pathological.

This is not to say that empirical issues are unimportant. Nor is it to say that general ethical principles are irrelevant. Rights and responsibilities, autonomy and beneficence, for example, have all been widely discussed in the literature (Macklin, 1982). But involuntary psychiatric treatment is a specifically *medical* intervention. Hence while there may be other grounds for, say, preventing someone from killing themselves (for example paternalistic or religious grounds), the grounds required for involuntary treatment are specifically medical. There is something about (certain forms of) mental illness that (for most people) justifies involuntary treatment, but it is not immediately clear either what this is or how it should be assessed. The practical need is thus not just for ethical clarification but for clarification specifically of the medical concepts of illness and disease.

Linguistic analysis

As a way of doing philosophy, linguistic analysis is a form of conceptual analysis. Philosophical problems, according to this approach, are, in part, illusions; they are problems, if not created, at least compounded by philosophers taking a too narrow or restricted view of the concepts with which they are concerned. What is required, then, in tackling such problems, is to find a better vantage point. This is provided by ordinary usage – that is to say, the uses of language in everyday, technical and non-technical, as distinct from merely philosophical, contexts. Hence the method of linguistic analysis is to look carefully and comprehensively at ordinary usage. There are dangers in this. In particular, ordinary usage often incorporates the very difficulties – the confusions and obscurities – with which philosophy should be concerned. Ordinary usage is thus not to be taken as, somehow, the measure of 'truth'. Rather it is a resource. It is a resource of linguistic data that can help to inform and fill out philosophical examination of the concepts in a given area of discourse (Austin, 1956–7).

The linguistic analytical approach can be helpful in medical philosophy at a number of points (Fulford, 1990). It may be used directly to explore the medical concepts, either in general or in particular areas of psychopathology. It may also be used indirectly as a way of examining the debate about these concepts in the literature. It is with the direct uses of linguistic analysis that we will be concerned in this section, returning to its indirect uses in the next. In both cases we will continue to have involuntary psychiatric treatment particularly in mind.

A philosophical version of the medical model has been widely adopted by both sides in the debate about mental illness. Thus opponents of the concept, noting that mental illness is a relatively value-laden concept, argue that only physical illness is a truly scientific and hence genuinely *medical* concept. This is the basis of Szasz's view that involuntary psychiatric treatment, even in the case of a suicidally depressed patient, is not really treatment at all, in the medical sense, but coercion reflecting social value judgements (Szasz, 1960).

Supporters of mental illness on the other hand, have reacted to such arguments by seeking to show that in the relevant respects it is indeed, like physical illness, a properly scientific concept. Among doctors, this is the line taken for example by Kendell (1975) and by Campbell (1979), both of whom argue that mental illness can be analysed like physical illness in terms of a value-free biological–scientific notion of impaired functioning. Similarly, Wing (1978), and more recently Roth and Kroll (1986), while emphasising the social context of medical practice, make this line of reasoning the basis of their respective justifications of involuntary psychiatric treatment. It is this line, too, which has generally been taken by philosophers interested in the medical concepts; Flew (1973), Glover (1970), and Boorse (1975), for example.

At first sight a science-based interpretation of the medical concepts is attractive. After all, scientific medicine has been highly successful. Hence in order to undermine the authority of medicine in a given area, as in respect of involuntary psychiatric treatment, it might seem to be sufficient to show only that what is being done in that area in the name of medicine is not in fact scientific. Equally, in order to defend the authority of medicine in that area, it might seem to be necessary only to show that it *is* scientific.

However, closer inspection of the ways in which the medical concepts are actually used suggests that this science-based view is at best one-sided. In emphasising the mainly factual connotations of the concept of physical illness, it is consistent with the way the concept is used in the context of the 'high tech' procedures that are characteristic of hospital medicine. But in other contexts, in primary care for example (Helman, 1981), and in lay or non-technical usage (Barondess, 1979), the concept of physical illness may be used with markedly evaluative connotations. This has been emphasised as much by sociologists as philosophers (Lockyer, 1981). What it suggests, however, is that at any rate beyond the bounds of hospital medicine, the medical concepts, physical as well as mental, are not purely scientific but in part evaluative in meaning.

It might still be thought that this is consistent with the standard view of medicine as essentially a science in its more technical aspects. Boorse (1975) is among those who have developed a medical model along these lines, distinguishing between theoretical (scientific) and practical (value-laden) uses of the medical concepts. We will be examining his arguments in the next section. First, however, we must consider an alternative move which is available to those who would retain a science-based view of medicine. This is to focus attention, not on the broad concepts of illness and disease, but on particular kinds of psychopathology.

It is this approach which has generally been adopted in relation to involuntary psychiatric treatment. It is a pertinent approach, given that such treatment is indeed largely confined to a particular group of mental disorders, the psychoses. These disorders, furthermore, seem particularly well suited to analysis in value-free scientific terms. Thus, corresponding as they do with the traditional 'insane', their characteristic feature is lack of insight. This is a difficult and indeed contentious psychopathological notion (David, 1990). But for practical purposes it can be equated with the presence of delusions; and delusions, so many authors, medical and philosophical, have argued, can be analysed in traditional scientific terms as, or as a product of, impaired cognitive functioning.

Such an analysis, if right, could do the work that is required of it in relation to involuntary treatment. Treatment of this kind, it will be recalled, requires specifically medical grounds; and the proposed analysis of delusions, in terms of impaired *functioning*, could provide such grounds. Further, the particular impairment of functioning that is suggested, impaired *cognitive* functioning, does indeed seem to be capable of justifying involuntary treatment at least in cases other than mental illness. Cognitive impairment underlies the justification of such treatment in cases of confusion, for example, and mental deficiency.

This raises a difficulty, however, namely that of specifying the particular kind of cognitive functioning that is involved in delusions. Delusions occur in a wide variety of mental disorders and in some of these, in dementia for example, there is cognitive impairment. But as yet no disturbance of cognitive functioning that is characteristic of delusions has been identified. The obvious response to this is that the nature of delusions – as false beliefs – points at least to *some* disturbance of cognitive functioning. Flew (1973) takes this line, for example. He points out that standard text-book definitions of delusion are in many respects unsatisfactory. Such definitions, in an attempt to mark out pathological from other kinds of false belief, usually suggest that delusions are culturally atypical (but many are not), incorrigible (but new ideas, for instance, have to be incorrigible to survive) and unfounded (but without further analysis this is question begging, and mere consensus won't do). Yet it remains the case that delusions are false beliefs, often bizarrely so. This falsity, then, suggests there must be some impairment of cognitive functioning which in principle could provide the justification for involuntary treatment. Indeed, Flew concludes, implicit in the falsity of delusions is an objective standard of verification which provides, as he puts it, the 'one sure defence' against the abuse of such treatment.

This looks like a bull's-eye, then, for the science-based view. However, it is here that the method of linguistic analysis is decisive. According to this method, it will be recalled, we should look carefully and comprehensively at the actual uses of our concepts. And when we do this for the concept of delusion we find that as symptoms of mental illness, delusions are not *essentially* false beliefs at all. That is to say, the standard text-book definition of delusion (as a false belief, etc.) correctly describes the most common kind of delusion occurring as a symptom of mental illness. This is no doubt why the symptom is called a delusion, since, in non-medical contexts, the term delusion is used simply of false beliefs. But in medical contexts, the standard text-book definition notwithstanding, the word delusion is used of other kinds of belief altogether. It is used, first, of true beliefs, not just of beliefs that are thought to be false and then turn out to be true – although these are well represented in the literature – but of beliefs that are known to be true all along. This is well recognised clinically as an exception to the text-book definition. In the Othello syndrome for example, the patient suffers delusions of infidelity. And as Vauhkonen (1968) and others have pointed out, whatever else the diagnosis of this condition depends on, it is not that the patient's beliefs are, as to the plain facts as it were, known to be false at the time the diagnosis is made.

Delusional true beliefs are relatively uncommon, it is true, though no less pertinent to our understanding of the clinical concept of delusion for that. Even less common, and yet still more pertinent, is the occasional (and on the standard definition, paradoxical) delusion of mental illness (Fulford, 1989, ch. 10)! On the other hand, relatively common – indeed clinically commonplace – are delusions that are not beliefs at all, at any rate as to matters of fact, but value-judgements (Fulford, 1991). These occur characteristically, though not only, in what are called the affective psychoses, both depressive and (with elevated mood) hypomanic. Thus in depression a delusion of guilt may take the form of a factual belief, that the patient is responsible for some major disaster, for instance. Equally, however, a delusion of guilt may take the form of a value-judgement (mixed forms are actually the norm). Thus one patient, having forgotten to give his children their pocket money, believed that this was 'the most wicked' thing he could have done; that as a result he was 'worthless' as a father; and that his family would be 'better off' if he were dead. Delusional value-judgements in hypomania, by contrast, are generally positive rather than negative in sign. They are not always moral, but may be for example aesthetic or self-aggrandising.

Delusional value-judgements, despite being clinically commonplace, are generally not marked out as such in the text-books. Delusions are classified medically according to content (guilt, grandiose ability, persecution and so forth) rather than by logical form. This is because, for any given condition, factual and evaluative delusions have identical implications for treatment. A depressed patient with delusions of guilt, for example, will be treated in the same way, including involuntary treatment where appropriate, regardless of whether the delusions in question are evaluative or factual. From a philosophical point of view this is a rather striking observation – that facts and values, ostensibly so different logically, should have identical implications. But from a medical point of view it means, simply, that there has been no reason to differentiate between them. The importance of the linguistic analytical method is thus emphasised, for the philosophically crucial observation, that delusions may take the form of value-judgements as well as statements of fact, is to be had only by direct inspection of ordinary medical usage.

The fact value distinction

There is a strong case for believing that better understanding of the logical relationship between facts and values is likely to be important in medicine. Consistently with the science-based view, much of the literature on the concepts of illness and disease has taken its inspiration more or less directly from the philosophy of science. But in many respects ethics is the more relevant discipline. Indeed the dispute in the medical literature about mental illness is no less than a *forme fruste* of the is–ought debate in ethics. As we saw earlier, the debate about mental illness is concerned with whether this ostensibly evaluative notion can be defined in purely scientific terms, as the notion of physical illness is supposed to be. The is–ought debate is concerned, similarly, with whether evaluative notions in general can ever be defined in terms that are value-free (Warnock, 1967).

The relevance of the is–ought debate to medicine can be illustrated by considering Boorse's (1975) version of the science-based view in more detail. As noted in the last section Boorse is among those who have sought to retain a science-based view of medicine while taking seriously the evaluative connotations of the medical concepts. He achieves this by drawing a distinction between theory and practice. Medical practice, he suggests, is indeed value-laden. But at the heart of medicine is an area of purely scientific theory. This area is made up of concepts defined, at base, in terms of impaired functioning. This notion, in turn, is 'continuous with theory in biology and the other natural sciences' and hence is value-free.

The attractions of this approach are evident enough. It secures the concept of mental illness against its critics. More importantly, as a science-based account, it provides in principle what Flew claimed for his objective account of delusions, namely a 'sure defence' against the abuse of psychiatric treatment for personal or political ends. Further, it does all this within the specifically medical grounds necessary for the justification of specifically medical interventions, as in the case of involuntary psychiatric treatment.

For all the advantages of this approach, however, Boorse's own use of the term disease suggests that his definition may not be soundly based. The key observation is that notwithstanding his proposed value-free definition of disease, he continues to use the term with definite evaluative connotations. For example, having defined disease in value-free terms as 'a *deviation* from the natural (= statistically typical) functional organisation of the species', just two lines later he writes of it in value-laden terms as 'a *deficiency* in the functional efficiency of the body' (1975, p. 59). Similarly, later on, although he claims to have given a value-free account of mental disease, he describes it in value-laden terms as an 'interference' with mental functioning (1975, p. 62). Of course, these could just be slips of the pen. But Boorse, after all, is writing carefully. Hence what they suggest is rather that, however strong the motive for seeking to define the medical concepts value-free, once they are so defined they become incapable of doing the work that is required of them in ordinary usage, whether theoretical – as in Boorse's case – or practical. In other words if disease is defined value-free it ceases to mean disease.

A possible way round this is provided by the ethical theory called moral descriptivism. The central claim of moral descriptivism is that at least some value-judgements are entailed by, and to this extent reducible to, matters of fact (Warnock, 1967). Given only the requisite facts, moral descriptivism claims, the relevant value-judgements follow by virtue solely of the meanings of the terms in which they are expressed. Interpreting the science-based approach as a descriptivist approach is thus, on the face of it, a way of having one's cake and eating it too. It allows what Boorse says he is after, a 'value-free science of health' (1975, p. 49). It allows this, however, not by excluding value but by reducing the relevant (medical) value-judgements to the requisite facts. Hence, since *ex hypothesi* the value-judgements are entailed by the facts, descriptivism also allows – what Boorse's account does not – continued use of the medical terms as value terms.

Moral descriptivism thus seems to offer all the advantages of a science-based account of the medical concepts while avoiding a major objection to it. Furthermore, when it comes to involuntary psychiatric treatment, descriptivism would seem to offer the further advantage of halving the difficulties of interpretation presented by the (key) clinical concept of delusion. For by holding out the prospect of reducing values to facts, it holds out the corresponding prospect of reducing evaluative delusions to factual delusions.

Descriptivism is very far from being universally accepted, however. Indeed, the majority of philosophers would probably agree with Hume in recognising a divide between fact and value, or at any rate between 'is' and 'ought'. There are wide differences of opinion as to what kind of a divide this is. Hare (1952) is a leading exponent of the non-descriptivist view that it is a logical divide. While stressing the mixed factual and evaluative nature of most terms in ordinary usage, he argues that it is always impossible, logically impossible, to define a genuinely evaluative notion in purely descriptive terms.

Non-descriptivism furthermore, has a number of implications which are helpful to our understanding of the medical concepts. In particular, it offers an explanation for the relatively value-laden nature of mental illness compared with physical illness. According to this approach, the relative strengths of the evaluative and descriptive connotations of a value term in a given context, is a reflection of the extent to which the descriptive criteria for the value-judgement expressed by that term are settled or agreed upon (Urmson, 1950). If there is much variation in the criteria the term will have mainly evaluative connotations (as in 'good picture'). If the criteria are largely settled the connotations will be mainly descriptive (as in 'good apple'). Hence, as against the science-based view, if illness is a value-term, mental illness is neither invalid because of its evaluative connotations nor in need of redefinition in purely descriptive terms. On the contrary, the difference between mental illness and physical illness in this respect emerges simply as a property that illness shares with value-terms in general.

In relation to delusions, on the other hand, non-descriptivism might seem at first glance an unpromising theory, and on just the points that descriptivism seems promising. Denying the reduction of values to facts, it doubles (where descriptivism halves) the difficulties of interpretation. Moreover, the very existence of delusional value-judgements could be taken as evidence against it. For in denying the reduction of values to facts, non-descriptivism has the consequence that any value-judgement is logically (though not always psychologically) possible. Yet here, apparently, in the clinical phenomenology of delusions, are to be found value-judgements which are not merely false, but false in a sense which is so close to that in which factual delusions are false that, as noted earlier, the two kinds of delusion have generally not been differentiated.

Closer inspection shows, however, that on both these points, non-descriptivism is on the contrary the more promising view. First, with regard to the difficulties of interpretation, the effect of non-descriptivism is not to double them but simply to bring us square on to their full extent. It could be, as descriptivism suggests, that delusional value-judgements are to be understood in terms of delusional factual beliefs – that is, by reduction of the former to the latter. This, indeed, is one possible explanation for their identical practical implications. But in itself, this tells us nothing at all about what it is for either variety to *be* a delusion. In particular, it says nothing about delusional true factual beliefs or the delusion of mental illness. On this account, as on conventional science-based accounts, these unusual, but logically crucial, species of delusion must be written off as mere oddities, pointing, at most, to some (as yet to be defined) disturbance of cognitive functioning.

Non-descriptivism, on the other hand, automatically incorporates – and can be extended to explain – the full (logical) range of delusional phenomenology. I have discussed this in detail elsewhere (Fulford, 1989, ch. 10). The key, however, is just that consequence of non-descriptivism which led to the second point on which it appeared unpromising, namely that any value-judgement is logically possible. Thus, granted this consequence, what follows from the existence of delusional value-judgements, according to non-descriptivism, is that *pathology* in value-judgements has to consist in something quite different from (or at any rate additional to) *logical* invalidity as such. This then leaves open the possibility that whatever this 'something' is, it is the same 'something' that *pathology* in factual beliefs consists in. And this possibility is consistent with the fact that delusional value-judgements and delusional factual beliefs have identical practical implications. Non-descriptivism thus provides an explanation for these identical implications which is quite different from that provided by descriptivism. Where descriptivism explains them by a (horizontal) reduction of evaluative delusions to factual delusions, non-descriptivism explains them by a (vertical) reduction of both to this 'something'. But non-descriptivism goes one better than descriptivism. For if pathology in factual beliefs is understood in this way, then the (still hypothetical) 'something' not only makes possible – and in this sense incorporates – but it actually predicts the existence of delusional true factual beliefs and, by analogy with the classical paradox of the liar, the delusion of mental illness.

To this extent then, non-descriptivism is indeed the more promising theory. It fits better. To take matters further, of course, the 'something' at the heart of the non-descriptivist account has to be fleshed out. Otherwise, better fit or not, non-descriptivism leaves us with no actual advance in understanding. This is how descriptivism left us, implying, yet being unable to put any flesh on, the corresponding notion at the heart of its account, that of impaired cognitive functioning. Again, I have gone into the non-descriptivist 'something' in more detail elsewhere (Fulford, 1989). It emerges from a non-descriptivist account of the medical concepts in which the actual experience of illness is interpreted in terms of its (logical) links with failure of action, in contrast to the logical links between disease and failure of function; and in which, correspondingly, delusions are interpreted in terms of defective reasons for action in contrast to impaired cognitive functioning. This amounts to a programme for, rather than a conclusion to, non-descriptivist work in this area. But as an account of delusions it is at least consistent with the full range of the clinical phenomenology of this remarkable symptom.

Conclusions

This chapter began with a reading of its title as a plea from those either weary of medical ethics or unpersuaded of its practical value – Oh no! *Not* more medical ethics! The argument having now run its course it may seem that we have ended up on a somewhat abstract plane. In fact though, we have been focusing, at ever-higher magnification, on the concepts implicit in involuntary psychiatric treatment: first on the concept of mental illness, with which the specifically medical ethical issues raised by such treatment are associated; next on the concept of delusion, the paradigm symptom of mental illness; and finally on the evaluative logical element in the concept of delusion as revealed by its clinical phenomenology. The whole process has thus been one of clarification. This has not as yet been taken very far. Even so, it has had the effect of underpinning the grounds of compulsory treatment by showing their essential coherence. It has also provided a framework of new ideas for future research directed towards better understanding of these grounds, with potential applications to the practical difficulties raised by marginal cases and by the misuses and abuses of involuntary treatment.

Conceptual analysis, as has been emphasised, is not the only approach which is required to tackle problems of this kind. General ethical issues are important, as are other disciplines – psychology, sociology, anthropology, biology. Furthermore, clarification of concepts can make life, or at any rate show it to be, even more complicated than it appears. In the present case, the fact/value distinction, useful as it may be, is itself highly contentious philosophically. And even to the extent that conceptual clarification is possible, it is no guarantee of better practice. In the absence of the impulse to act ethically, clarification may be used as readily for the purpose of bad practice as of good. But for all this, clarification is a condition of better practice wherever medical decisions turn not on the acquisition of the facts but on the construction that is placed on them. To this extent therefore, conceptual analysis could make a specifically philosophical contribution to the day-to-day practice of medicine, generating not *more* medical ethics, but a more *medical* ethics.

ACKNOWLEDGEMENTS

I am grateful to Dr Grant Gillett, Mrs Caroline Miles and Dr Janet Soskice for their helpful suggestions during the preparation of this chapter.

REFERENCES

Austin, J. L. (1956–7) 'A plea for excuses'. *Proceedings of the Aristotelian Society*, 57: 1–30. Reprinted in White, A. R. (ed.) (1968) *The Philosophy of Action*. Oxford University Press

Barondess, J. A. (1979) 'Disease and illness – a crucial distinction'. *The American Journal of Medicine*, 66: 375–6

Bloch, S. (1981) 'The political misuse of psychiatry in the Soviet Union'. Ch. 18 in Bloch, S. and Chodoff, P. (1991) *Psychiatric Ethics* (second edition). Oxford University Press

Boorse, C. (1975) 'On the distinction between disease and illness'. *Philosophy and Public Affairs*, 5: 49–68

Campbell, E. J., Scadding, J. G. and Roberts, R. S. (1979) 'The concept of disease'. *British Medical Journal*, 2: 757–62

David, A. S. (1990) 'Insight and psychosis'. *British Journal of Psychiatry*, 156: 798–808

Flew, A. (1973) *Crime or Disease?* New York: Barnes and Noble

Foucault, M. (1973) *Madness and Civilization: A History of Insanity in The Age of Reason*. New York: Random House

Fulford, K. W. M. (1989) *Moral Theory and Medical Practice*. Cambridge University Press

(1990) 'Philosophy and medicine: the Oxford connection'. *British Journal of Psychiatry*, 157: 111–15

(1991) 'Evaluative delusions: their significance for philosophy and psychiatry'. *British Journal of Psychiatry*, 159: 108–12, supplement 14, Delusions and Reality

Glover, J. (1970) *Responsibility*. London: Routledge and Kegan Paul

Hare, R. M. (1952) *The Language of Morals*. Oxford University Press

Helman, C. G. (1981) 'Disease versus illness in general practice'. *Journal of the Royal College of Practitioners*, 230 (3): 548–52

Kendell, R. E. (1975) 'The concept of disease and its implications for psychiatry'. *British Journal of Psychiatry*, 127: 305–15

Lockyer, D. (1981) *Symptoms and Illness: The Cognitive Organization of Disorder*. London and New York: Tavistock Publications

Macklin, R. (1982) 'Refusal of psychiatric treatment: autonomy, competence, and paternalism'. Ch. 6 in R. B. Edwards (ed.) *Psychiatry and Ethics: Insanity, Rational Autonomy, and Mental Health Care*, 331–40

McGarry, L. and Chodoff, P. (1981) 'The ethics of involuntary hospitalization. Ch. 11 in Bloch, S. and Chodoff, P. (eds.) *Psychiatric Ethics*. Oxford University Press

Roth, M. and Kroll, J. (1986) *The Reality of Mental Illness*. Cambridge University Press

Szasz, T. S. (1960) 'The myth of mental illness'. *American Psychologist*, 15: 113–18 (1963) *Law, Liberty and Psychiatry: An Inquiry Into the Social Uses of Mental Health Practices*. New York: Macmillan

Urmson, J. O. (1950) 'On grading'. *Mind*, 59: 145–69

Vauhkonen, K. (1968) *On the Pathogenesis of Morbid Jealousy, with Special Reference to the Personality Traits of and Interaction between Jealous Patients and their Spouses*. Copenhagen: Munksgaard

Warnock, G. J. (1967) *Contemporary Moral Philosophy*. London and Basingstoke: The Macmillan Press Ltd

Wing, J. K. (1978) *Reasoning about Madness*. Oxford University Press

Index